Ready, S

M000309477

THE

DAD'S GUIDE

TO

PREGNANCY

WEEK BY WEEK

Preparing *First Time Dads*
for fatherhood through tips and tricks,
decoding doctor visits and being a
reliable support system for your
partner.

*Confidently become the Dad you want
to be!*

AARON EDKINS & MEGHAN PARKES

Are You Ready to Be A Dad?

P *ush as if you are taking the biggest crap of your life!"*

A sentence I can honestly say I have never heard before. Especially not from a medical professional and certainly not one directed at my wife.

But, doctors' orders, right?

My wife continues to push, she has been pushing for over three hours now.

In front of me, I stare at this woman who I have known for much of my adolescent life and cannot fathom how she is still working through this. The look of determination in her steely eyes cannot be replicated and can only be applauded. I would have given up hours ago. Waved my white flag and asked to rain check this for a later date.

The phone rings in the delivery room; the nurse sneaks a look of concern at the doctor and whispers in her ear. I already don't feel right about this.

"We will have to consider other options. The baby's in distress. We can try forceps or a vacuum to help maneuver the baby out. We may have to perform a c-section if neither methods are successful."

I steadily recall the reading I've done on forceps and vacuums; there are some safety concerns but are generally considered safe. Maybe we should go this route? Luckily, this is done in my head and not out loud. It appears my wife is feeling drastically different about it.

She shoots me a similar look as the nurse, though this one isn't concern or fear. It is a sincere intent. She squeezes my hand even tighter, and I swear I feel the bones in my knuckles grinding together. My wife screams through clenched teeth, "this baby's coming out on its own free will, and I'll be damned if they interfere!"

I know this woman, despite never seeing this look before. She means what she says.

As she bears down on the bed, I hold her knee up to her ears while simultaneously rewetting a rag for her forehead.

The room counts to three in unison. It seems we are all gritting our teeth now. We're all bearing down.

"STOP PUSHING! THE HEAD IS CROWNING."

They begin to prepare for the baby to make its arrival by placing a blue tarp on the floor. I start panicking that the tarp is there in case they don't catch the baby. Then I quickly recall this is to saturate all the blood and fluids that will soon be overflowing from baby's release.

The rest is a blur. I now realize I have never indeed known love before. I've never truly appreciated my wife as sincerely as I do now. The amount of love in that room could have filled a football field twice over.

After nine months of doctor appointments, shuffling through baby names, and counting from four to forty weeks - the time had come. I couldn't recall the last time I waited nearly a year for such a life-changing event.

"Hey, Dad! Over here!" yells the nurse, which snaps me back to the present.

I look around half expecting a brawny good-looking man to walk over with heightened confidence that picks the baby up with one hand in Heisman stance. But no stud comes and there is no one handed-pick-up, we've missed out on the football pose.

My mind eventually shifts into gear to the sudden realization of my new title.

"Wait a minute, that's me, I'm the dad!" (still, a stud of course) ... Then, with unwavering focus and extreme precaution, I gently cradle the baby in my two arms. My baby.

Filled with extreme happiness, I stare in disbelief at my newborn son and make a silent promise never to disappoint him. At that very moment, no words could describe my feelings of jubilation and honor and I could not feel more proud or excited for what the rest of life has to offer for my family and me, for the three of us.

So ... how did I get here? ... And, how can you be ready for this moment?

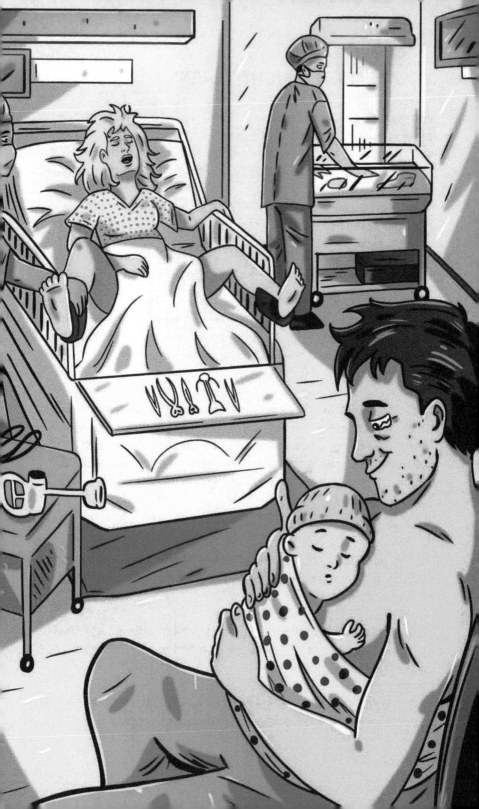

YOU'RE ON THE RIGHT TRACK!

You may be picking up this book the day you heard your partner is expecting, or you may be in the middle of the pregnancy and realize you're not as prepared as you would've hoped, or you may not even be a dad yet, but you want to understand what to expect in advance.

Wherever you are on this quest – Congratulations! You are taking the necessary steps to educate yourself and be serious and proactive about pregnancy and fatherhood.

YOUR JOURNEY

The journey you have ahead of you will be the most incredible experience of your life. Bigger, better, and more exciting than anything you can imagine. To be filled with many highs, some lows, and a ton of uncertainty.

There are things you may already know, many you want to know, and an endless stream of things you don't know. Whether it be reviewing what to ask during a hospital tour to decoding what blood test results mean to just knowing that as a father-to-be, we need to step up, be supportive and present throughout the process.

MY BIGGEST REGRET

As the old saying goes, "Women become Mothers the moment they find out they are pregnant, but Men become Fathers the first time they hold their children in their arms."

As a general rule, this cannot ring any truer for most males. Looking back, I feel as though this perfectly summed up my first experience of pregnancy.

To this day, I continuously feel as though I could have done more to support my partner. Through each subsequent pregnancy, I made a valiant effort to devote myself to my partner as she was devoting herself to creating our growing baby.

Now, as a father of three, after realizing my lack of education on pregnancy the first time around and not understanding how to adequately support mom, this was certainly my biggest regret.

I believed the pregnancy was happening to her since she was growing the baby. That my job started at intercourse and ended with conception and I was furloughed, benched if you will, until I needed to tap in again once the baby was born.

Lesson learned - be more emotionally connected and physically involved and don't let your partner tackle the next nine months feeling alone.

I'm here to tell you that you don't need to make the same mistakes and it is a simple fix through knowledge and preparation.

WHICH SEAT DO YOU CHOOSE?

In just the first few weeks, a mother has front row seats to watch her body change from weight gain and stretch marks, fear of the unknown impending of childbirth, and a mindset that has been severely altered and clouded with pregnancy hormones.

Your partner will change physically, emotionally, and mentally. During this time, some men can't help but position themselves in the backseat. We are not the ones being poked at during weekly doctor visits, we (more or less) remain the same clothing size, our energy and resources aren't shared with another being, and we certainly have no idea what it's like for a baby to kick from deep within our bellies.

Taking the backseat approach is not a bad thing. But what if men could ride up front instead? Close enough to their partner to be in the moment with them, and near enough to not just go through the motions but be part of them?

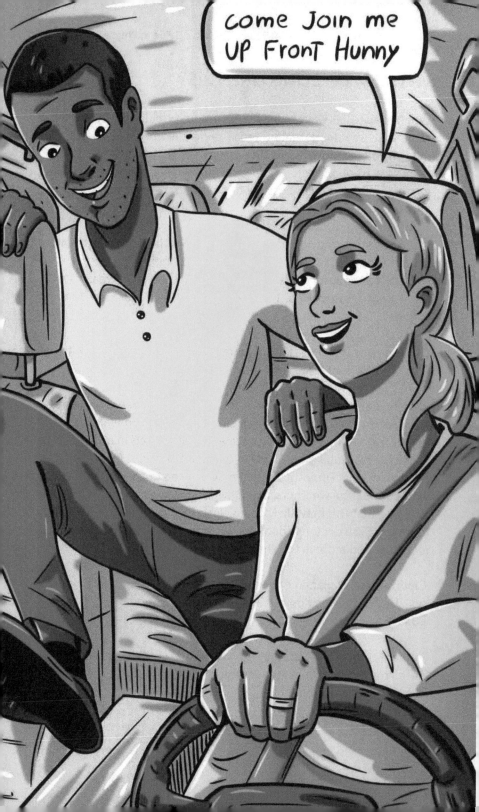

WHY AM I FEELING LIKE THIS?

When my partner was pregnant with our first child, I downloaded the same apps she did, attended those same child birthing classes, and read through countless blogs. I noticed that I needed various resources to obtain information, but they were all geared towards women. It felt nearly impossible to find solid material from the male perspective.

On top of this, I had no one to confide in over the first three months. My partner and I chose to follow the superstitious rule that you shouldn't announce your pregnancy until after twelve weeks due to the risks of a miscarriage. This made me feel even more isolated and helpless.

Of the few resources I did find, rarely did they cover the emotional roller coaster I was experiencing.

Whilst, many soon-to-be Dad's feel an uncontainable amount of anticipation and joy to meet their child, it's also reasonable for many to feel anxious and unsure. On a scale, your emotions may range from anxiety to jubilation, fear to confidence, loneliness to companionship. For instance, you may be used to Tuesday date night with your partner or Thursday night poker games with your friends. Realizing that this may likely change can be overwhelming and scary for many. Each doctor's appointment that you attend, may make you feel more and more in the shadows.

A lot of these similar emotions are shared by the soon-to-be mom as well. However, men don't tend to talk about it as openly or freely as women.

I'm here to reassure you that it's ok to have all these thoughts and feel all these different emotions, you are not alone, I certainly felt the same!

YOUR PREGNANCY CONFIDANT

You may be asking, what prompted me to write this book? Well, as the first person out of my brothers, cousins, and friends to have a baby, I casually fell into the role of "pregnancy confidant" or "the go-to-guy for when shit hits the fan". After a friend has upset their nine-month pregnant partner by telling them they don't understand why she's so tired - I can expect a call and a solution for their problem. What starts as a quick call for a not-so-quick answer, turns into a full-blown conversation with daily check ins. I provide support for others, normalizing their experiences and concerns, and have been a dependable resource for those around me embarking on the uncharted territories of pregnancy.

THE GO-TO PREGNANCY HANDBOOK

Throughout this book, you will discover how your baby is developing, symptoms your partner may be feeling, and how you as a father can navigate these nine months. Each of these information-packed chapters is at your disposal through easy to follow weekly guides. Because how much time do we really have while preparing for a baby?! We need to get all the date nights and poker tournaments in while we still have the chance!

Filled with helpful tips and ideas on the best ways you can get involved and actively contribute towards the pregnancy, while providing support and encouragement for mom. We'll also cover a wide range of topics from basic reminders to major discussion points including researching parental leave, finding a suitable pediatrician and budgeting for baby now and in the future.

Three children later, and I find myself referring back to my notes in this book. You may find the same occurs for you as well. Balancing work commitments and/or becoming wrapped up in your growing children, leaves little room for remembering the to-do lists and special reminders.

READY, SET … PREGNANT!   The Dad's Guide to Pregnancy

Pro Tip:	If you have to ask your partner if she needs a foot massage, you're already too late!

Consider this your go-to pregnancy handbook.

THE OUTCOME

At the end of the nine months, not only will you have a profoundly appreciative partner that will be eternally grateful for your love, support, and understanding, but you will also be better prepared for your new baby's arrival!

There's no better time than now. It's time to step up, be proactive, and drop the "dude" bravado. You are the role model your child will see every day. Be the best version.

Roll up your sleeves, throw out any excuses, and let's get down to business.

And remember, you are in this together.

So, let's get started …

HOW TO USE THIS BOOK

I would suggest reading this book from start to finish to get an overall grasp and understanding of what lies ahead and then revisiting each week as you follow along your partner's pregnancy.

Alternatively, for those that may have time constraints or perhaps are less avid book readers, simply follow along the weekly guides to stay on top of things!

Glossary Section:	There is also a helpful glossary at the end of the book with useful pregnancy related terms. Whilst reading, if you come across any unfamiliar words, flip to the glossary at the back of the book for a full list of simple definitions.

Additionally, during each week of the pregnancy journey you will be presented with the following 4 weekly icons, which represent:

✓ Baby's developmental updates

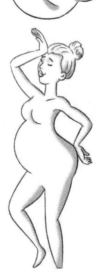

✓ Changes with mom
both physically and emotionally

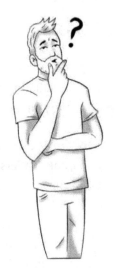

✓ Feelings and thoughts you
   may experience

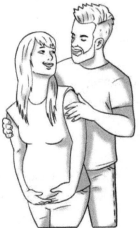

✓ Ways you can stay actively
   involved and show support for
   mom-to-be

(Please note, these icons will only appear when there are new updates from the previous week)

WHAT DO WE COVER?

We focus on the 9-month period from falling pregnant (conception) to the birth of your baby.

Note – we do not cover information on how to successfully conceive (or fertility) and we only cover the essentials for after birth (postpartum). If you would like further informational guides, please check out the rest of our pregnancy and parenting book series.

STEERING YOUR WAY THROUGH THE WEEKLY PREGNANCY GUIDE

Introduction:

Are You Ready To Be A Dad?

Opening Comments

Chapters are divided into manageable weekly blocks as shown on the next page:

PART 1 - Buckle Up, We're Heading Into The First Trimester

Chapter 4:   MONTH 4   WEEKS 14-17

PART 2 - Second Trimester: The "Honeymoon Period"

Let's Paint the Picture: *Protecting the Bump*

Chapter 5:   MONTH 5   WEEKS 18-21

Let's Paint the Picture: *Revealing Baby's Gender*

PART 3 - Third Trimester: The Final Countdown!

PART 4 - Labor, Delivery and Postpartum Essentials: Let's Get Ready To Rumble!

Conclusion:

Now You're Ready To Be A Dad!

Appendix

DISCLAIMERS

We acknowledge that there's so much information out there in the form of books, internet, phone apps, social media platforms, articles, blog posts and so on. Our goal is to present to you a simplified version of everything you need to know, broken down into easy to digest and manageable bite size weeks.

Think of this book as a convenient compilation of information and reference materials, appropriately organized in one place. It is structured in a logical and helpful order, that is easy to follow along and presented in an entertaining way.

At times throughout the book you may encounter certain information is repeated, but rest assured this is to emphasize the importance of particular points and to help stay on top of essential reminders.

Please note the information contained within this document is for educational and entertainment purposes only. All effort has been executed to present accurate, up to date, reliable, and complete information, however no warranties of any kind are declared or implied. Readers acknowledge that the author and publisher is not engaging in the rendering of legal, financial, medical or other professional advice of any kind. Readers should consult a licensed professional before attempting any techniques outlined in this book. The strategies and general advice in this book are not always suitable for every person and the reader is advised to do their own research to assess its suitability to their own circumstances. The content within this book has been derived from various sources and all warranties are strictly disclaimed without any exception.

By reading the contents of this book, the reader agrees that under no circumstances is the author nor the publisher responsible for any damages or losses, direct or indirect, or any adverse circumstances arising from the application of the books contents, which are incurred as a result of the use of the information contained within this document, including, but not limited to, — errors, omissions, changes or inaccuracies. Whilst this book contains information and quotes from individuals, institutions, organizations, government bodies and websites, readers should be aware that neither the author nor publisher specifically endorses any of the entities referenced. Additionally, some websites may have dissolved or changed from the time of writing this book to when it is published or read.

PHYSICAL AND EMOTIONAL CHECK INS

As everyone's bodies and emotions are different, the symptoms and feelings experienced throughout pregnancy can greatly vary. Each person will have a unique journey and encounter different levels and severity of symptoms which may be felt at different times throughout pregnancy. The symptoms mentioned throughout this book are a reference guide only, and it is expected that they may vary for each individual. However, as always if you suspect something is not right, then please consult your professional medical practitioner for further advice.

PRENATAL & POSTPARTUM DEPRESSION

Many men and women experience postpartum depression with overwhelming feelings of sadness and many choose to keep these feelings to themselves (especially men). If you are experiencing severe anxiety, stress or loneliness during or after pregnancy, be sure to speak to your doctor for a confidential chat. If you are not ready for this conversation, there are other preliminary measures you can find online called "prenatal or postpartum depression quizzes". Remember you are never alone and someone will always be there, you just need to find the courage to reach out.

Please refer to the Resources section for some helpful links.

MISCARRIAGE AWARENESS

A miscarriage is when your baby (embryo or fetus) doesn't survive before 20 weeks of pregnancy. This can occur for a number of reasons such as:

- Problems with chromosomes that would prohibit normal fetal development
- Hormone imbalances from mom
- Moms age, a higher risk if over 35 years old

This loss is incredibly difficult for both mom and dad. The most common feelings are guilt, anger, and sadness towards the loss of the baby.

If you experience a miscarriage during the pregnancy, reach out for professional help and know you are not alone.

Please refer to the Resources section for some helpful links.

OTHER BOOKS IN THE SERIES

In partnership with my co-author Meghan Parkes, keep an eye out for additional books we will be adding to this pregnancy and parenting series over time.

The next instalment of the "Ready, Set ..." series covering your '*Baby's First Year*' will be out soon!

If you would like to join our mailing list to be notified of new release books, simply email me at edkinsbooks@gmail.com.

In the meantime, check out Meghan's latest pregnancy book –

'40 Things You Must Do, Before You're Due!'

(First Time Moms Pregnancy Guide)

– It's one helluva read!

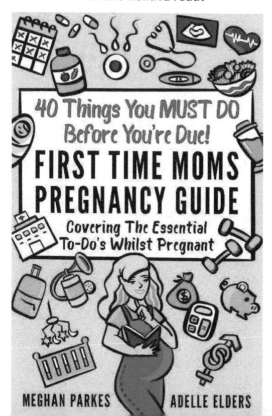

FEEDBACK

Both Meghan and I would really appreciate your feedback and thoughts on the book. We welcome any positive comments or even any possible suggestions to improve the book for future editions. Please, don't be shy, let us know your thoughts at: edkinsbooks@gmail.com

Part 1 - Buckle Up, We're Heading Into The First Trimester
(Includes Weeks 1 through 13)

MONTH 1 - Weeks 1 through 4
Learn about:

+ **Ovulation:** *the best time to get down to business* - now is when we morph into jackrabbits

+ **Conception:** *did all our hard work pay off?* - should we re-morph?

+ **Implantation:** *the fun side of science* - bound to test your patience.

+ **First Doctor's Visit:** *and what the heck it all means* - HCG, what?

Let's Paint the Picture:
Trying to Conceive

Back row of the movie theater: done
Restroom at Arbys: done
Passenger seat of my mom's minivan: done

We couldn't keep our hands off each other. We were sex-driven rabbits who kept things interesting. No place was off limits and no time was inconvenient for us.

Fast forward to five years later. My wife shared that she wanted to start trying to have a baby, I didn't blink an eye or question her. I knew exactly what had to be done. The same thing we were doing for years and years before.

But after six months, I found myself bored with the activity. You see, it wasn't the sex that turned me off. It was the strict schedule.

If my wife was ovulating, then I knew that the entire week we needed to have sex at least once a day. Sex was followed by my wife rushing me off so she could throw her legs up in the air. She heard this would help trap the sperm and persuade it to connect with her eggs.

Well, you can forget Arby's restrooms. There's certainly no room to throw your legs up in there.

This is a very common occurrence when couples start trying to conceive. It tends to start as fun and exciting, a quest that couples are more than happy to achieve. But the longer the process takes, the quicker they can lose interest and it may start beginning to feel like a chore.

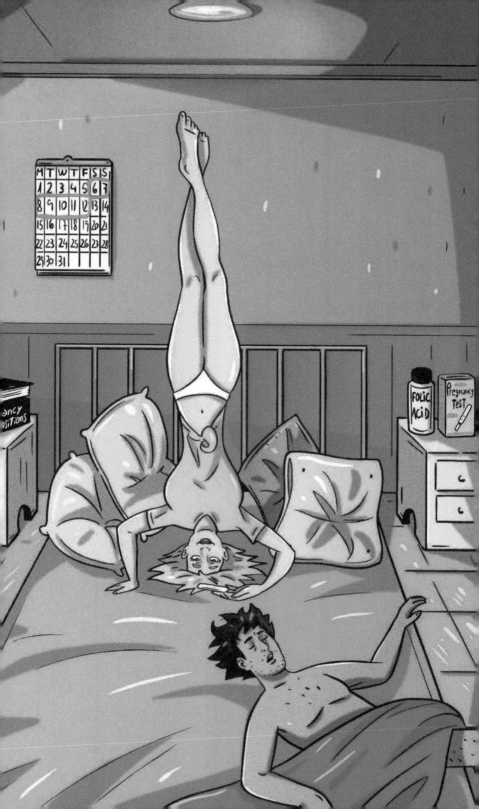

For Weeks 1 and 2 we will cover this process a bit more in-depth, so we fully understand the science behind it all. We will also review how to keep the process enjoyable, as well as potential reasons why conception may not be successful.

Welcome to Week 1
Pregnancy Preparation:
'One Week Pregnant' But No Baby?

<u>TL, DR (or 'The Short Version')</u> : *Before falling pregnant it's important to plan ahead.*

4 minute read

Fast facts covering :

- One week pregnant - what does it mean?
- Conversations with your partner
- Difficulties conceiving

One week pregnant refers to the time before your partner ovulates (releases her egg/s). She is currently on her period and not yet pregnant. So while she is not actually pregnant, this week is still counted in the total 40-week countdown.

Starting in week 2, you will begin to try and conceive, as this is the time your partner is most likely ovulating. This is the time where your sperm and her eggs join together. Fast forward to week 4 or 5 where we will find out if the meeting was successful!

Let's talk about sex, baby. Let's talk about you and me.

Salt-N-Peppa had the right idea. Now is such an exciting time full of possibilities for you and your partner. This is the best time to have an open discussion on both of your expectations.

Agreeing to have a baby is at times a pretty lengthy conversation. What may start as a simple "should we, shouldn't we" usually leads to religious views, political opinions, family input and ends with how everyday life will quickly change. These are important topics to address so it is best to do so as openly and honestly as possible from the start.

Each of these items is guaranteed to come up at least once during the pregnancy, and certainly through your child's life. Let's get all of the elephants out of the room before conception. :: trumpet sound::

Difficulties conceiving - Am I shooting blanks?

Becoming pregnant may take a couple of tries or could take months or years. Either time frame is totally normal and depends on each individual.

Other than sheer timing and frequency there are many reasons conception may not work. It can be an underlying issue with the female or male. The most common are:

Heads Up:	Exercise caution discussing these with your partner. You are just asking to have a shoe thrown at your head. Instead, it is best to get checked by a healthcare provider to rule out any concerns.

Female:

- **Age (Over 35 or Premature Menopause)** - Many couples are not ready to have a baby until later in life but due to the shifts in a woman's hormones as she ages, this can lower the chances of conceiving. On top of this added pressure to beat the clock, the pregnancy is now considered "high risk" which means your partner's (or baby's) chances for health complications or preterm (early) delivery increase.

- **Endometriosis & Polycystic Ovary Syndrome (PCOS)** –are two common conditions affecting your partner's ability to conceive.

Reminder:	Refer to the Glossary Section at the back of the book for a full range of pregnancy related definitions.

Male:

- **Low Sperm Count** - You may have some strong fighters that you're shipping off, but if there aren't enough of them it may not take. The more sperm, the better. It simply increases your chances to conceive. It is recommended you have a semen analysis to test your levels.

Pro Tip:	**Test your sperm count** - A semen analysis is a very effective and easy test... Masturbate in a cup and proudly walk over to the nurse to hand off your 'mini-yous'.

Week 1 Dad's Guide

Baby's Development
- Non-existent!
- But in the weeks ahead, you'll see your baby go from a pin to a soccer ball!

Mom's Changes

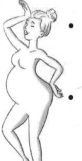

Physically:
- May experience changes in vaginal discharge. During ovulation, she will release discharge that helps make sperm more hospitable when meeting her eggs.
- Possible bloating and/or lower back pain

Emotionally:

- Since this is after your partner's menstrual cycle, she may be feeling good as the outlook of having a baby is in her grasp.
- However, it's also possible for hormone changes to cause mood swings and headaches.

Dad's Feelings

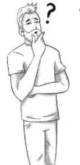

- Thoughts of reality may start to set in. By having an open conversation about the future, it starts to make things very real. Embrace these feelings and pat yourself on the back for considering all possibilities.

Supporting Mom

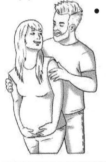

- Now is the time to cut out any adverse habits such as smoking and drinking. Both can be a stress reliever, so without them - she may be feeling a bit out of whack. The good news is, she will probably sleep better and think more clearly. You may want to consider cutting these habits out as well in solidarity.

Pro Tip:	Encourage foods rich in folic acid such as leafy green vegetables, citrus fruits and legumes, as they significantly reduce baby's risk of developmental defects by 70-80%.

Pro Tip:	**Healthy Habits!** - Exercise, a healthy diet and a regular sleeping routine are all essential for your partner when trying to fall pregnant. Suggest a regular exercise routine to do together, keep track of your weekly progress and consider going bed together at a set time each night.

Welcome to Week 2
Intimacy: *It's Business Time!*

TL, DR: *YouTube search - Flight of the Conchords: Business Time (3:44 version)*

5 minute read

Fast facts covering :

- The last day of your partner's menstrual cycle
- The chances of successful conception
- Keeping sex enjoyable
- Practicing patience

We've reached the last day of your partner's menstrual cycle. Time to get down to business, take the sheet off the ghost, hold nothing back, go for the Full Monty... "I know what you're trying to say... You're trying to say it's time for business, It's business time, ohhh" (if you haven't heard the song "Business Time by Flight of the Conchords", you should give it a listen)

Note:	The journey to becoming pregnant can actually take much much longer. Until we know if your sperm has joined your partner's egg, we will carry on with the idea that it was successful. If not, do not fret, it is called a journey for a reason.

Timing is EVERYTHING! What are your chances of success?

The best way to increase your chances is to have sex as often as you can close to the time your partner is ovulating. Remember the more sex you have, the more likely you are to conceive but this needs to be done at the right time as well. How do you know the right time? Check with your partner first. She may be tracking this pretty closely.

Once your partner's period is over, she starts ovulating and her egg(s) are now available for your sperm to fertilize. Your partner's egg may be released anytime over a 12-14 day span and it's normally available for only up to 24 hours for fertilization, therefore regular sexual intercourse is a must!

Sex becomes a chore? This must be a typo...

Sure, washing your car is enjoyable. But what if you washed your car twice a day, every day for 7-10 days straight? The novelty begins to wear off. Heck, the paint may start to wear off.

I won't sit here and tell you to make each time special and unique. It just isn't possible. We've only got so many tricks up our sleeves. The main thing to remember is to enjoy your time together and not take it too seriously. Some suggestions are role-playing, music selection, change of location, varied time of day, etc.

So, remember... if you have to wash your car a bunch of times, at least put on some really good music and switch up your motions. *Wax on, wax off anyone?*

Pro Tip:	It's important for you both to be relaxed as possible when having intercourse, so have a fun night in (or out) and try to forget that you're trying!

What's the ETA on the results?

Oh, how I wish this was a quick and precise response. You *may* be able to tell within the next two weeks after a trip to the doctor (we will cover this more during Weeks 3 and 4). This all depends on when conception actually occurred which can take anywhere from

3-5 days.

Now is the time to *'woosa'* and wait it out!

This is one of those times that I wish I could tell you that by the second or third child the waiting process gets easier… It doesn't. It gets worse because you already know what to expect from the pregnancy, but you're not sure when you should start preparing until it's confirmed.

Week 2 Dad's Guide

Baby's Development

- Bueller Bueller… that's right, still nothing yet!

Mom's Changes

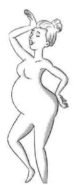

Physically:

- Increased sex drive. Great! We will need this to finish strong.
- Similar symptoms to week one

Emotionally:

- Mom might be feeling some anxiety. She isn't sure if conception has occurred which means she might not be sure how to feel just yet.
- Similar symptoms to week one

Dad's Feelings

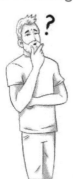

- Pretty in line with mom. This similar feeling between you and your partner may not last long as the pregnancy progresses, so use this time to relate with one another.
- Enjoying the intimacy!

37

Supporting Mom

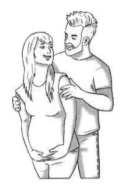

- Remind her that while there is only so much the two of you can do, now it is up to the sperm and egg to make things happen. Keep things light. Oh, and keep having lots of sex. If that's not support, I'm not sure what is.

Did You Know?	**Cut down on caffeine -** When trying to fall pregnant and once your partner is pregnant, experts recommended that mom limits her coffee (or caffeine) intake to one cup per day.

Fun Fact:	**Did You Say Twins?** The probability of having twins is considerably higher if your partner is over 35 years old! This is due to the fact that she is more likely to release more than 1 egg during ovulation.

Welcome to Week 3
Quality Time Together:
Calm Before the Storm

TL, DR: *Relax & enjoy time together before the at-home pregnancy results next week (week 4)*

3 minute read

Fast facts covering :

- Calculating due dates
- Enjoy your time together

Due Dates: Will your baby be born on the due date?

Not likely. It is pretty rare for babies to be born at the exact 40-week mark. This is because calculating a due date is pretty tricky. Unless you conceived through IVF (which has an exact date of implantation). The due date should be referred to as the "Estimated Due Date."

Fun Fact:	The due date is calculated from the first day of your partner's last period. However, due dates are not an exact science and are usually wrong by almost 99%!

Bonding with your Partner: Just the Two of Us

Have you ever heard the saying "calm before the storm"? This is what week 3 is reserved for. It is the time after all the lovemaking and before the many doctor's visits. In two short weeks, you will find out if this duo will soon become a trio (or quartet).

Have a few recipes you've been wanting to try? Use this time to have a fun cooking day together. Sure, it may not be Michelin Star, but it will be edible and it will be enjoyable!

Week 3 Dad's Guide

Baby's Development

- There are around 250-300 million sperm every time you ejaculate! When you ejaculate inside your partner, only 1 sperm will survive the 10-12 hour voyage and make it to successfully fertilize your partners egg! The fertilized egg is technically called a "zygote" cell. This zygote cell gradually splits into hundreds of smaller cells and embed themselves into mom's uterine wall lining, which later form the baby embryo and placenta!

Did You Know?	It is your sperm that determines your baby's gender which happens now at conception, but normally you won't find that out until around 16-18 weeks.

Mom's Changes

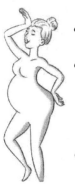

Physically:
- Mom may be feeling no symptoms at all, yet. This is totally normal.
- Some moms may feel tummy cramping, breast tenderness, and even a heightened sense of smell. (Keep the beef jerky sticks at a clear distance)

Emotionally:
- Most women experience a mix of anxiousness and excitement during this time.

Dad's Feelings

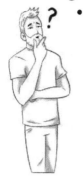

- You may still be very much in line with mom's feelings. Similar to weeks 1 and 2, use this time to bond and openly share your feelings.

Supporting Mom

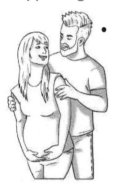

- As the results are still unknown it's best that you both stay busy and keep your mind off the impending confirmation of your baby. Enjoy your time together before the true excitement sets in. Surprise mom with a fancy night out on the town, dinner at your favorite restaurant, a spa day, or even cooking a meal at home together.

Welcome to Week 4

Home Pregnancy Test:
Is Your Bun In The Oven?

TL, DR: *Possible confirmation that your buns in the oven!*

5 minute read

Fast facts covering:

- At-Home Pregnancy Test
- Preparing for the first doctor's visit
- Self-Care

Implantation occurs during week 4 and in simple terms, it's when the embryo attaches to your partner's uterus wall and begins to grow. Once there has been successful implantation, you may be able to take an at-home pregnancy test.

Couples usually take the at-home pregnancy test in either weeks 4 or 5. Some may see positive results as early as 4 weeks after conception and the most common reasons for this are they may either be further along than they thought or their HCG levels are high enough to detect it. (*For definitions, refer to the Glossary section at the back of the book*).

Your chances of seeing the most accurate result are to take the pregnancy test after your partner has had a missed period. It will also help to select a test that guarantees a 99% accuracy rate. That's right, not all tests are created equal!

Pro Tip:	If you had a positive test, congratulations! If it was negative but your partner still thinks she is pregnant,

> then schedule that first doctor or midwife's appointment so you can 100% confirm the potentially exciting news!

First Doctors Appointment - What to expect?

The first visit usually occurs next week (Week 5) to allow enough time for the HCG levels in your partner's blood to reveal a positive or negative result.

Your doctor may also decide to perform a transvaginal ultrasound as well. This is an exciting time for mom and dad as you are able to get a front-row seat to your growing little speck that will soon be a bouncing baby! You may also see the amniotic sac which is where your baby will live and grow! This forms about 12 days after becoming pregnant.

Other than the bloodwork and ultrasound, you can also use this time to ask the doctor for anything you should be doing in the meantime. For example, is there a certain prenatal vitamin your partner should be taking? Should she take it easy for a bit? Use this time to learn as much as you can from the doctor before your next visit.

Did someone say "Self-Care Sunday"?

You heard right.

This week is all about self-care for you and your partner. Why not kick it off with a nice group workout? Exercise can be overwhelming for some and calming for others. Focus on trying to make this an enjoyable experience for you both.

No need to perform shuttle sprints at full tilt! Simply walking around the block or a gentle swim are great ways to keep the body moving and in shape while your partner prepares for the baby.

Discussion Point:	**Move Or Improve?** – Is your current housing situation suitable for your new family member? Is there adequate space? Or you may find your current situation is perfect and only requires minor tweaks!

Week 4 Dad's Guide

Baby's Development

Size Estimate:

- Eye of a sewing needle – (dad by day, seamstress by night)
- The bunch of cells has now settled in mom's uterine wall lining, where it will remain for the next 8 months until birth. The cells have now also split into two parts.
- One half being the embryo (or soon-to-be baby) and the other half is the placenta which is where your baby will obtain all their oxygen and nutrients from mom and secrete waste until birth.
- Baby's organs are now under construction!

Mom's Changes

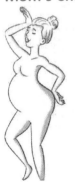

Physically:

- PMS type symptoms and cramping are typical at this stage
- Possible increase in breast tenderness and sensitivity
- Frequent urination could be an early indicator of a successful pregnancy

Emotionally:

- If there was a positive test, mom is most likely in shock. It's all starting to come together!

Dad's Feelings

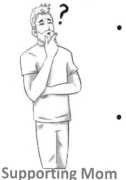

- If there is a positive test, you're probably feeling the excitement. It worked. All of your palling around in bed these past few weeks has paid off. You made a baby. WOW. Take a moment to really take that in.
- The next 6-8 weeks are especially crucial to the development of your baby.

Supporting Mom

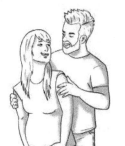

- Make a promise to yourself that you will be an active part of this pregnancy. One of the best ways, is to start attending as many doctor appointments as possible. You will not regret it. Plus, it will provide her some support for debriefing each visit.
- Take it a step further and jot down questions before each appointment. It will mean the world to her that you took the time to do so and shows you're fully invested in the process. The next appointment will be in week 5.

Twin Pregnancies:	By the end of Week 4, there will be two embryos, each with their own placenta and amniotic sacs.

Month 1 Checklist & Reminders
(Because who has time to make their own list?)

☐ Discuss your plans for the future with your partner

☐ Have tons of sex (especially around ovulation)

☐ Step away from the booze and smokes

☐ Make your first doctor's appointment (Week 5 and Week 8)

☐ Relax and rejoice in the happy news

☐ Eat a healthy diet and exercise frequently

MONTH 2 - Weeks 5 through 8
Learn about:

- **First Doctors Visit:** *pregnancy confirmation after the at-home test*

- **Pregnancy Hormones**: *your partner's experiencing a ton of changes*

- **Baby's Heartbeat**: *now detectable!*

- **First Prenatal Visit**: a *comprehensive look at baby*

- **Heightened Sense of Smell**: *mom's new superpower!*

Let's Paint the Picture:
Hormone Changes

I could feel her staring at me from across the table. I looked up, we made eye contact, and I smiled. She smiled back but I could tell something was bothering her. This has been the third day in a row that my wife hasn't sat near me during a meal. I spent the previous night racking my brain on what I could have done wrong.

It was Monday night and I made our favorite dish: Meatless Monday Taco Bowls. On any other week, she would have fought me for the last scoop of homemade guac and beer-battered chips. No, I don't mean she would have slid her spoon into the bowl and gently scooped. Yes, I mean she would have put the spoon to my throat and used her bare hand to scoop the said guac and chips. But that was my wife. Never afraid to order the biggest meal or finish her dish before anyone else. One of the many things I adored about her. Who knew the day would come when I'd long for food fights with her.

"Hunny, um, is everything alright? Do you want some extra chips?", I ask her through legit hesitation. *"Does it look like I want chips?"*, she replies sharply.

After an awkward meal of her moving food around her plate and me chewing as softly as possible, we head to bed. I start my research on alien abductions and begin to make a game plan. And then it hits me. An alien didn't take my wife, she's still there.

She just has some new *qualities* about her that happened to spring up right around the time we found out we were pregnant. We are officially eight weeks pregnant now.

I make a note to myself to switch up our usual meals and instead, ask her what she would like to eat. That seems a safer bet.

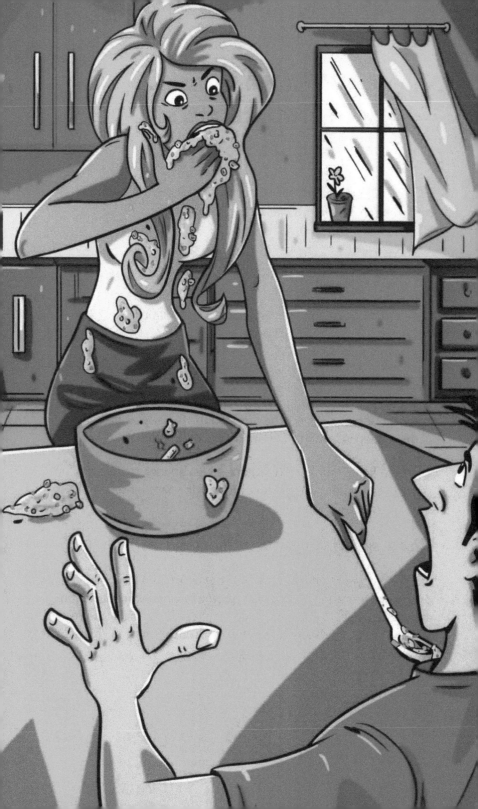

Welcome to Week 5
First Doctors Visit:
Shit Just Got Real!

TL, DR: *1-2 days to get blood tests back for pregnancy confirmation* and *mom's diet may increase*

3 minute read

Fast facts covering :

- First Doctor's Visit - Pregnancy Confirmation?
- Eating for two - fact or myth?

Well, hello hello month two! This week you should be meeting with your OB GYN or midwife for the first time as a couple who is possibly expecting a baby! The pregnancy test was positive, so the blood work should reflect the same right? As we reviewed in Week 4, this all depends on how far along you really are.

Here's to hoping those HCG levels are high enough to detect! If not, come back in another 1-2 weeks after taking another test to see if the results have changed.

First scan: Will I see our bun in the oven?

At this visit, your doctor will be able to confirm the at-home pregnancy test after running your partner's blood work. It can take anywhere from 1-2 days to get the results back. Sit tight, the results will be in soon. And remember, you can't do anything to change them.

Eating for Two - Should We? Shouldn't We?

Now, this is a tricky myth to bust. I'll share with you the truth, and then I'll share with you what you should share with your wife.

THE TRUTH: Mom does not physically need to eat for two in order for your baby to develop properly. In fact, a woman does not need to consume any additional calories until the second trimester which should only be about 340 more each day. This goes up slightly in the third trimester to 450 calories.

Heads Up:	To put this into perspective, 340 calories is the equivalent of about two Guinness Draught beers.

SAFE TO SHARE: Mom can eat whatever she wants, whenever she wants. If she wants an extra bagel to kick off the day, simply slide your plate over and let her have it.

Week 5 Dad's Guide

Baby's Development

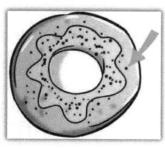

Size Estimate:
- Poppy Seed (Fun Fact: the poppy seeds on that tasty bagel can actually return a positive drug test!)
- Big changes for your baby's major organs including the heart, stomach, liver, and kidneys.
- Let's not forget digestive, circulatory and nervous system developments
- Baby's heart will start beating and they will start resembling a mini tadpole with a tiny head and small tail.

51

Mom's Changes

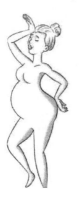

Physically:
- While it may be hard not to comment on them, mom's breasts may slowly start growing. Along with this new development, there may be some sensitivity and soreness associated with it.
- So for now, hands off the merchandise.

Emotionally:
- Mom is most likely feeling pretty drained. This can carry on from now until the second trimester, so if she expresses the need for a nap - be sure to fluff the pillows.

Important:	If your partner is taking medication, have them reviewed by her healthcare professional to double check they're safe to continue using.

Supporting Mom

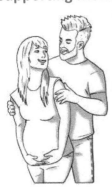

- Take the lead and schedule the first prenatal visit. It will be one last thing for your partner to check off the never-ending to-do list. The next is week 8.
- Since mom has a new role to play as mother, take over household chores that she would usually do especially the manual, labour intensive ones. Prioritise most important to least and encourage her to relax as much as possible.

Pro Tip:	Be sure to attend all appointments and remember even questions you may think are bad, will be looked upon favorably because you're making an effort!

Welcome to Week 6
Houston, We Have a Heartbeat!

TL, DR: *Baby's first developmental milestone & Mom's hormones are rapidly changing.*

5 minute read

Fast facts covering :

- Baby's heartbeat - *possibly* detectable between weeks 6-8
- How pregnancy hormones affect your partner

One small leap for Dad, one giant leap for baby!

You read that correctly. Your tiny growing baby now has a heartbeat and has reached their first developmental milestone! Baby's heart rate can range from 100-150 bpm (nearly twice as fast as an adult) and will continue getting faster over time.

It may now be detectable via ultrasound but hold onto your patience for just a bit longer, as it is normally heard anywhere from Week 8-10. If you can't hear it, don't worry, you may not be as far along as you thought.

Pregnancy Hormones & Your Partner

Around this time is when a shift may occur with mom. This is primarily due to the pregnancy hormones that are causing your partner to not quite feel like herself. For example, pre-pregnancy she may have been able to stay up late at night without falling asleep mid-show. Or maybe she could have gone an entire car ride to the mall without three bathroom breaks. Whatever it may be, these are things of the past, so be ready to support and embrace the new changes for a while. Having said that, some may struggle to relate to what she is feeling or the changes she is experiencing, which can cause a little disconnect between the both of you.

I say, bridge the disconnect now. Get on the same page as your partner, and express that while you may not have the swollen breasts or extreme fatigue, you're in this together and will support her from now through the rest of this pregnancy.

Week 6 Dad's Guide

Baby's Development

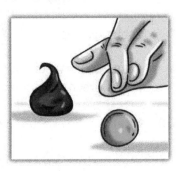

Size Estimate:

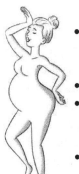

- Delicious Chocolate Chip Morsel or Green Pea (guess which one your partner is probably craving)
- Since it's so awesome, let's give props to that heartbeat one more time!
- Though it may be difficult to imagine, week 6 is just the start of your baby's face beginning to form. This includes the cheeks, chin, and jaw! Buds will also start forming, which eventually become arms & legs

Mom's Changes

Physically:
- Morning Sickness (nausea and vomiting) rears its ugly head and it sticks around for a while. (Heads Up: it should be called "anytime-of-day-sickness").
- Increased breast tenderness from Week 5.
- Regular bathroom visits for urination are likely to persist .

Emotionally:
- Overall fatigue is still very much present and maybe taking a toll on mom.

- Your partner has a large influx of hormones running through her body that she may not have ever experienced before. This may cause her to be overly tired, moody, and a bit sensitive.

Dad's Feelings

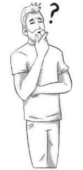

- You may feel a bit of guilt while seeing mom go through so many emotional changes
- These are totally valid feelings that some dads may not immediately share with their partner, but I encourage you to always maintain open and honest communication with her.

Supporting Mom

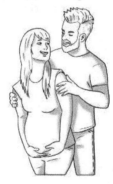

- Show your support by listening to her if she wants to discuss these symptoms. If she doesn't bring them up, be sure to check in to see how she is feeling at least once a day.

Heads Up:	**Cat owners** - Ensure your partner does not empty the kitty litter box as cat feces can cause serious harm to the unborn baby. This goes for the entirety of her pregnancy. Also avoid uncooked or raw meats (including fish) as this can affect your baby in a similar way.

Welcome to Week 7
Smell: *Mom's New Superpower!*

TL, DR: *Help your partner through nausea & possibly her new "Super Smell Sensitivity"*

4 minute read

Fast facts covering :

- Mom's heightened smell sensitivity
- Keeping mom comfortable and hydrated

Mom's (Not-So-Fun) New Superpower

Normally around weeks 7 and 8, your partner may be experiencing her "super smell sensitivity!" This might seem kind of fun… cool even. Sure, it is pretty great if she is smelling flowers or perfume, or maybe even just being out in the fresh air.

Alas, this is not the case here. She may be way more likely to pick up ill odors than pleasant ones. So that means, any unbearable smells around the house that have the slightest odor, will need to go otherwise this can induce vomiting and an overall uneasy feeling for mom. Think expired food, dirty smelly clothes, old shoes lying around, and even unwashed pets!

Get to it before her "spidey senses" beat you to it!

Staying hydrated!

Whether that lovely woman carrying your child is your partner, your wife, your best friend, your video-game buddy - she needs your support this week as nausea takes on a whole new form. A once usually happy, calm, and collected woman may start showing a different side to herself due to this symptom as well as extreme fatigue.

Now is the time to really step it up. Try to recall your last hangover. Sucked, right? You couldn't keep food down, smells set you off and you forgot to drink that water despite it being next to your bed. Times that by about ten, then add a growing baby inside you.

One easy way to help here is to remind her to continuously drink water. Water hydration helps mom's body absorb nutrients, which ultimately feeds through to your baby. There are great mobile apps out there that can send drink reminders in a subtle way. You may want to take the liberty of downloading this for her. Another easy idea would be getting her a creative water bottle. Popular ones include sayings every few ounces as encouragement, such as: "way to go", "almost done, "you got this, mom!"

Pro Tip:	According to Healthline.com - "Taking a combination of Unisom and Vitamin B-6 is one remedy that some doctors recommend to help women deal with morning sickness" *(As always, please consult your doctor regarding the suitability of any types of supplements, as they may vary from person to person).*

Fun Activity: Gender Guessing Game

- Chinese Gender Predictor (google it) - relies on dates of conception
- Mom's skin glowing - Boy for yes, girl if not
- Mom craving sweets - Boy for yes, girl for savory
- Beats per minute for baby's heart - over 140 boy, under 140 girl

These may turn out totally wrong, but it's a bit of fun!

Week 7 Dad's Guide

Baby's Development

Size Estimate:

- Dice (better dust these off now before you're too tired to party)
- Baby has doubled in size since last week.
- What could be more fun than doubling in size? What about a set of kidneys? Baby is developing this major organ during week 7.

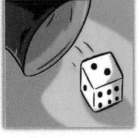

Did You Know?	The umbilical cord has now formed connecting baby to the placenta. Food and oxygen can now be transported from mom to baby and baby's waste is also transported back to mom via this cord.

Mom's Changes

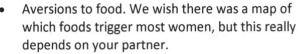

Physically:

- Sensitivity to certain smells that she may have enjoyed prior to pregnancy.
- Aversions to food. We wish there was a map of which foods trigger most women, but this really depends on your partner.
- Prepare to have a lot of interrupted meals and activities for bathroom breaks.

Emotionally:

- Mood swings are still coming in hot this week. Expect this one to stick around for at least a few more weeks.

MONTH 3 - Weeks 9 through 13
Learn about:

+ **Bonding with Baby**: *connect with your baby from deep inside the womb*

+ **First Trimester Screening**: *scheduling and preparing like a pro*

+ **Combating Moms Symptoms**: *increasing water intake*

+ **The Placenta**: *how to maintain the placenta with healthy eating*

+ **Mom's Increased Sex Drive:** *the moment we've all been waiting for*

Let's Paint the Picture:
Bonding in Today's Modern Age

To my beautiful baby,

I decided to write to you, my baby, every week starting right at that first positive pregnancy test. I didn't wait for the doctor's confirmation, either. As soon as mom showed me the proof, I felt like your Dad already. So, I started thinking -

How can I bond with you, before I meet you?

Your mom has a pregnancy journal called a "Belly Book" that she writes in after every doctor visit. Well, I don't have a belly (one that has a baby in it at least), but I do have a laptop and things I'd like to say to you.

That was how your email account came to be: "dadsnumber1fan@gmail.com". What? Well, I thought it was catchy and rolled off the tongue, no?

So far I've sent you twelve emails. Each with fun facts about myself and your mom, hopes for the future, and random conversations we've had regarding raising you. You'd be surprised about how much you can argue about whether or not to use a sound machine. *I vote yes.*

The doctor tells us that in just a few short weeks, I might be able to feel you kick. I'm really looking forward to that. Maybe you'll be the next Ronaldo.

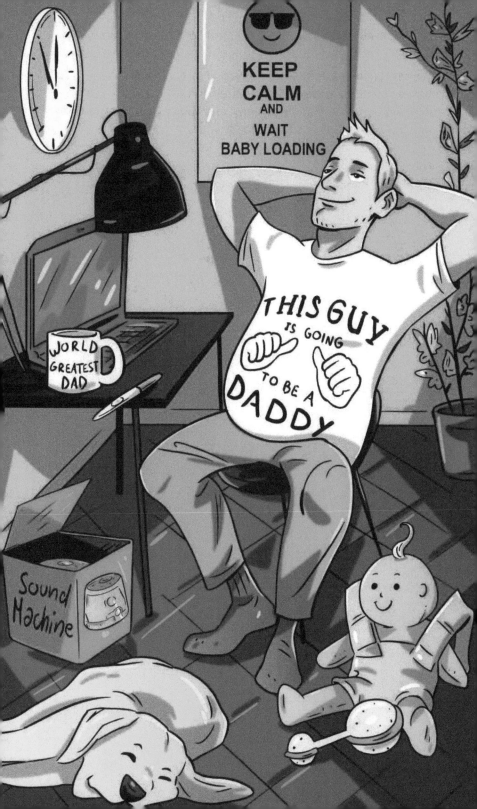

We're anxiously awaiting your arrival and I can't wait to meet you. When you're older we will sit together and review all of these emails. I hope you find them funny, and I hope you do become my number one fan because I'm already yours.

Love,
Your (Super Cool) Dad

Welcome to Week 9
Baby Bonding:
The Name's Bond, Baby Bond

TL, DR: *Tips to start connecting with your baby & now they are officially a fetus!*

4 minute read

Fast facts covering :

- Ways to bond with your baby
- Feeling your baby kick (or not)
- Baby's new developmental milestone!

So far you may feel like you're watching a movie from the outside, through a blackened window, without any sound. You're experiencing everything second hand based on what your partner shares with you and the short glimpse at your baby through an ultrasound. This can cause dads to begin to feel left out and potentially opt for that backseat role I mentioned earlier on.

Climb into the passenger seat, hold your partner's hand, and connect with your baby. There are various ways you can go about making this connection, I'll list a couple out for you:

- Start an email account for baby and send personal messages to them for you to review when they are older
  - o Write down what hopes and dreams you have for your child and the ways you will help achieve them
  - o Sending letters and messages to your baby will eventually be one of your most precious possessions, and I'm sure it will also become one of theirs.

- Talk and sing to your baby. Have a favorite song you can't get out of your head? Start singing to your baby and soon they will begin to recognize and feel comfortable with your voice and who knows, it may be their hit song one day too!

Can I feel my baby kick now?

Remember those webbed fingers and toes we talked about last week? They have just started moving around. No doubt practicing for when they need to swat at their crib mobile and rattle!

You won't be able to feel all of these movements and neither will mom. First kicks are usually felt closer to the second trimester. For now, just imagine how cute your baby looks doing water aerobics.

Developmental Milestone! Your precious embryo that started at the earliest stage of human development is now a fetus! This change officially happens at 11 weeks after your partner's last period or the 9th week after the egg has been fertilized.

Week 9 Dad's Guide

Baby's Development

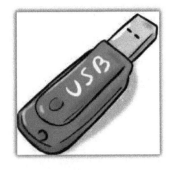

Size Estimate:
- USB Memory Stick (like the new floppy disc)
- Your baby has all the essential body parts and is starting to resemble a tiny human!
- Baby will start developing around 20 "baby teeth" buds, which are the ones that fall out during early childhood.

Mom's Changes

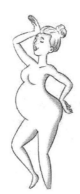

Physically:
New Symptoms:
- Mom may start experiencing the ever-popular... headaches, migraines, mind pains - whatever you call it, they are no fun.

Recurring Symptoms:
- Regular bathroom visits for urination and vomiting are likely to continue.

Emotionally:
- Mom may be feeling a bit defeated by the influx of pregnancy hormones that have hit her in just a few short weeks.

Dad's Feelings

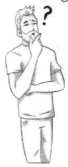

- Spending time to bond with your baby may create new feelings of connection as you start to imagine and picture life with your new baby. Thinking of your aspirations, hopes and dreams for your baby can help you start establishing an emotional attachment to them.

Supporting Mom

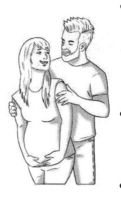

- Headaches aren't fun for anyone. Consider planning a relaxing day for mom during week 9. Think candlelit baths and soothing music. Barry White or John Legend, anyone? Don't worry, she can't get pregnant twice...
- Buy mom a journal to take notes of her daily or weekly thoughts during pregnancy. She may even want to fill it with messages for baby for when they are older!
- Double-check that the 12 Week prenatal appointment is booked

Welcome to Week 10
NIPT Testing:
Gender Reveal Already?

TL, DR: *Optional blood testing can reveal down syndrome & baby's sex, and mom may need a new outfit for her growing bump!*

5 minute read

Fast facts covering :

- First Trimester Testing & Gender Reveal …already!?
- Mom's Growing Belly

If you added up the number of times you've seen the doctor over the past year, it may not come close to the frequency in which you will be going now. I like to think pregnancy is shared between mom, dad, baby, and their doctor. They are there every step of the way. In fact, you won't go longer than a month without seeing them. When you reach thirty-six weeks, it becomes once a week. That's right. Once a week. Kind of like a *really* needy in-law…

Blood Tests for Down Syndrome & Baby's Sex (Optional)

'NIPT' (Non-invasive prenatal test) normally occurs around weeks 10-14 and is an *optional* pain-free non-invasive blood test, which checks for abnormalities such as Down Syndrome. At this point, the blood test can also be used to reveal your baby's gender, but don't get too excited yet, as it could take up to 2 weeks to receive the results. *(also refer to 'NT Scan' in Glossary)*

Week 10 Dad's Guide

Baby's Development

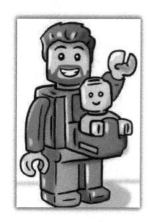

Size Estimate:
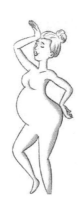
- Lego Man (these will soon be an everyday staple for you)
- Wondering what color eyes your baby has? Well, you won't find that out for a while and even if you could peek inside, your baby has their eyes closed until about 26-28 weeks.

Fun Fact:	Baby's brain is developing and their head accounts for roughly 50% of their entire body size.

Mom's Changes

Physically:
New Symptoms:
- Generally, around Week 10 is when women begin to display their small baby bump and can possibly experience belly pains and bloating as it stretches for baby.
- Constipation may rear its head, which can be helped with increased water and fiber intake.

Recurring Symptoms:
- Regular bathroom visits, Morning Sickness.

Emotionally:
- Due to the extra weight gain and new belly, it may have mom feeling frustrated with what she can actually wear. Her regular clothes may be

too tight, but she doesn't feel ready for maternity clothes.

Dad's Feelings

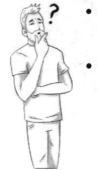

- There may be some nervousness about the upcoming first-trimester screening. This is a big test that will reveal a lot of information.
- As your partner begins to show, most men start feeling the gravity and realness of pregnancy. You may start having feelings of the need to protect mom's precious bump from accidental knocks when you're out and about and you may also feel a strong sense of pride that you are now a soon-to-be dad!

Supporting Mom

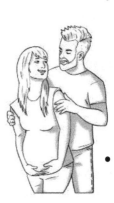

- If mom is starting to show already, she'll be needing some maternity clothes around this time and for the rest of the pregnancy. Make this a fun and memorable experience for her and take her shopping! She will rely on you for your thoughts since she has not shopped in this section previously. Another idea is to ask family and friends if they have any maternity clothes lying around that they are not using.
- Use this time to gather your medical records so you can provide the doctor with the most accurate information of both your family medical history and any conditions suffered.
- If constipation occurs, be sure to encourage fibrous foods such as fruits and vegetables and to stay hydrated by drinking plenty of water.

Welcome to Week 11
H2O: *Mom's Magical Potion On Tap! (literally)*

TL, DR: *Drinking water regularly helps alleviate some of mom's pregnancy pains.*

4 minute read

Fast facts covering :

- Water consumption during pregnancy

Water, Water, the magical drink …

I get it. Watching your partner going through all these new symptoms is not easy. Well, while we can't do much to help her ever-expanding bust line, we can help in other ways.

First, let's address those symptoms which can be relieved:

- Fatigue
- Leg cramps
- Itchy Belly and Skin
- Heartburn
- Swollen Feet & Ankles
- Headaches
- Insomnia
- Constipation
- Braxton Hicks
- Diarrhea

And now for the solution:

- Plain old H_2O

Mom's recommended intake throughout pregnancy is 8-12 glasses daily. Before you rush to her with this genius cure, keep in mind this will only help relieve the symptoms but not fully stop them. The best approach here would be to offer to increase your water intake with her. Be a sport, it's a team effort!

Oh, and when you both need to pee ten times as often, let her go first. Trust me.

Did You Know?	Dehydration can actually trigger mom to go into early labor, putting baby's health at risk. Another reason to ensure mom's water bottle is refilled throughout the day and start the good habits early on!

Week 11 Dad's Guide

Baby's Development

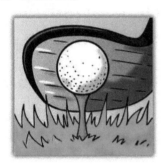

Size Estimate:
- Golf Ball (remember the good old days of last-minute golf outings?)

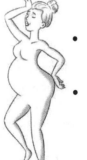

- Hair follicles are forming all over baby
- Nail Beds are forming which will soon develop into the finger and toenails
  - No, mom can't get scratched by the baby in the womb
  - Yes, you should purchase baby nail clippers
- The duck-like webbed hands and feet will start separating into individual fingers and toes.

Mom's Changes

Physically:
New Symptoms:
- An increase in appetite could signal the start of a gradual decline of mom's morning sickness!

Recurring Symptoms:
- Frequent urination, bloating, and constipation.

Emotionally:

- As you near the 12-week mark, many believe it is the safest time to announce your pregnancy because the chances of a miscarriage drop significantly from around 20-25% to less than 5%.
- Due to this, mom may be feeling excited to share her baby secret with more people. It is also common for this to feel a little scary as well. Once the news is out, it feels more real!

Dad's Feelings

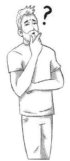

- Similar to mom's emotions. Itching to finally share the good news. (Just another week to go!)
- If you need some extra support or advice, you can reach out to friends of family that have been through pregnancy before. Ask them about their experiences and tell them about yours.

Supporting Mom

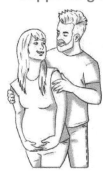

- You may have heard by now that pregnant women shouldn't lift heavy objects. If you see your partner carrying groceries or bringing in large packages - be sure to lend a helping hand.
- Encourage and motivate your partner to exercise, perhaps schedule a regular joint exercise routine together.

Pro Tip:	Prenatal Yoga has been shown to boost mom's mental health during pregnancy and foster feelings of calmness and relaxation.

Welcome to Week 12 Protecting Baby's Life Support & Sharing The News!

_TL, DR__: Mom needs to ensure she's eating healthy till birth to maintain the placenta and it is generally now safe to tell family and friends._

4 minute read

Fast facts covering :

- The importance of nutrition to mom & baby
- Sharing your baby news!

Can you believe there are only two more weeks until the second trimester? You are nearly a third of the way there. Give yourself a pat on the back for a job well done by keeping it cool and supporting mom and baby.

Want to know who else is supporting your baby? The placenta! This organ acts as your baby's critical life support by providing oxygen and nutrients and removing waste from your baby's blood.

Therefore, it is incredibly important that your partner sticks to a healthy diet while pregnant. This doesn't mean she can't indulge and enjoy the not-so-ideal foods at times. But at least the majority of consumption should be healthy. Eg. Vegetables, fruits, nuts, grains ...etc...and of course, plenty of water!

A reminder, the best way to think of this is if your baby was with you now - would you be feeding them those chips or cookies?

Fun Activity: Sharing The Baby News

Congratulations! You've reached Week 12 which means you are in what is generally considered as the "safe zone" (ie. significantly reduced risk of miscarriage) to share the news of your expected bundle of joy!

Let's talk about some creative ways to share the good news:

- Gathering friends and family for a photo but instead, make it a video where on the count of three you announce that you're pregnant! The footage will be priceless!
- Gifting a box with an item inside resembling your baby's size comparison and watch them guess what it means
- Present friends with a bottle of alcohol complete with a message that states "save this for me, we'll join you on *insert due date*" or (my favorite) add the same message from baby, with the date 21 years from now!
- Sending loved ones the ultrasound picture
- Or try googling - pregnancy chalkboard for mom and dad

Pro Tip:	Now is a great time to let your boss know as well. This will give them plenty of notice for your impending leave, allowing them to prepare replacement staff to cover your position well in advance.

Week 12 Dad's Guide

Baby's Development

Size Estimate:

- Toy Soldier (A good soldier never leaves a man behind!)

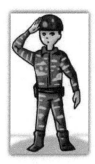

- All of your baby's organs are formed, now they will just need to continue to grow and develop.
- Baby is starting to open and close their fingers and curl their toes!
  - Hot Tip: if you poke your partner's belly during an ultrasound, your baby may respond back with a reflex.

Mom's Changes

Physically:
New Symptoms:

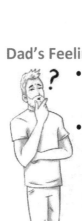

- Most women will start to show between now and 14 weeks if you haven't started already.
- Around week 12, many women notice some symptoms start to fade away including - nausea, food aversion, tiredness, breast sensitivity, and frequent urination.
- Mom may experience dizziness due to an increase in blood flow to the baby and less to mom.
- Unlikely to feel any movements from baby yet as they are still too small.

Recurring Symptoms:
- Bloating, constipation, smell sensitivity.

Emotionally:
- Mom may be feeling pretty hopeful and energetic! She may even be starting to feel like herself again with some relief from all the symptoms affecting her everyday activities.

Dad's Feelings

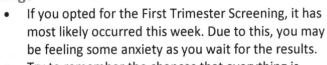

- If you opted for the First Trimester Screening, it has most likely occurred this week. Due to this, you may be feeling some anxiety as you wait for the results.
- Try to remember the chances that everything is okay should outweigh any anxious feelings.

Supporting Mom

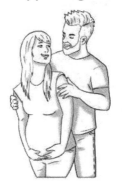

- As pregnancy hormones begin to fade away, this is the perfect week to start introducing weekly massages. At the end of each week, set aside some time for your partner to fully relax with a massage from you! This weekly ritual is sure to make mom incredibly happy, as well as, give her something calming to look forward to whilst enjoying some bonding time (also as a warm introduction to next week's discussion topic!).

Pro Tip:	If mom is experiencing tiredness, one possible solution is a regular carb intake and exercising to get the blood flowing around the body. On the other hand, sometimes all she may need to recharge those batteries is a good days rest, so pick up household chores and errands to give her a well-deserved break!

Reminder:	if your partner is struggling to keep down large meals, then suggest trying eating more smaller meals throughout the day. Bland or plain foods might be the new go-to and ginger infused drinks or foods will also help with any nausea.

Welcome to Week 13

Increased Sex Drive:
"When I Get That Feeling, I Want, Sexual Healing"

TL, DR: *A reduction in some of mom's pregnancy symptoms & week 2 "Business Time" is back on!*

5 minute read

Fast facts covering:

- Less hormonal symptoms for mom can lead to more interest in sex!
- Advantages of pregnancy sex

Maybe it's been weeks, maybe it's been months, maybe it's been days (you sly dog, you). Either way, sexy time might become a recurring event for you and your partner. In fact, around weeks 13-15, there may be an increase in your partner's sex drive. It is most likely caused by a reduction of some annoying pregnancy symptoms including less fatigue and nausea.

I'm sure you're wondering if you can poke the baby… I get it, Ron Jeremy, fair question. Allow me to put your mind at ease. Your penis cannot reach the baby. No matter how well-endowed you may be! Sorry, Ron.

Benefits of Pregnancy Sex (Other than the obvious)

Apart from being enjoyable, there are endless benefits to having sex with your partner while she is pregnant. Be sure to make her aware of these :

- Easing pregnancy aches and pains
- Enhancing both your moods
- Improving sleep
- Promotes bonding between the two of you
- It has also been known to help mom experience a speedier recovery after childbirth!

Week 13 Dad's Guide

Baby's Development

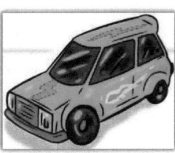

Size Estimate:

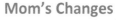

- Matchbox Car (or Hot Wheels, whatever strikes your fancy)
- Tiny fingerprints are now taking form, along with vocal cords!
- While you can't hear baby's sweet (and loud) noises inside the womb, you will definitely make up for lost time once your baby is born.
- At around 13 weeks, most babies start developing at different speeds, so keep this in mind for the remainder of the nine months.

Mom's Changes

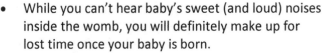

Physically:
New Symptoms:

- Increased sex drive (WOOHOO!)
- Mom's breasts will start producing the nutrient-dense "colostrum" (breast milk) in preparation for baby's arrival.

Recurring Symptoms:
- Frequent urination, bloating, and constipation

Emotionally:
- Moms newfound increase in energy is new this week and may continue on throughout the second trimester, which is why they call the second trimester the "Honeymoon Period". Let the good times roll!

Dad's Feelings

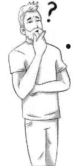

- With mom's new potential sex drive and energy boost, you are most likely feeling a little frisky and very happy with these developments!

Supporting Mom

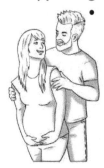

- **Pregnancy Pillow:** To ensure mom's comfort and baby's safety, your partner may start sleeping on her side. Surprise her with this thoughtful gift before she even asks. Yes, she can absolutely prop up a few bed pillows and place one between her legs at night, but trust me, this will be her new best friend providing her with ultimate comfort!

Twin Pregnancies:	If having twins, mom's bump will start to show a lot sooner, causing her to look further along in her pregnancy compared to a singleton pregnancy!

Month 3 Checklist & Reminders

(Because who has time to make their own list?)

☐ Make time to connect with baby

☐ Put together family history and medical records

☐ Schedule NIPT testing between 10-13 weeks (if you feel it is necessary)

☐ Get creative with baby announcements then share the news

☐ Starting at week 12, begin to schedule doctor appointments every four weeks

    ☐ 16 weeks will be the next one, then week 20 and so on

    ☐ During the week 20 appointment, there will be the usual prenatal appointment along with an Anatomy Screening

☐ Encourage your partner to drink more water

☐ Focus on a healthy diet and regular exercise routine

☐ Pick up some baby nail clippers

Part 2 - Second Trimester: The "Honeymoon Period"
(Includes Weeks 14 through 26)

MONTH 4 - Weeks 14 through 17
Learn about:

- **Planning your Babymoon**: *time for a romantic getaway*

- **Financially Planning for Baby**: *let's get those expenses in order*

- **Baby Can Hear You Now**: *speak up, your baby is listening*

- **Protecting The Bump**: *get on the defense and help guard moms growing belly*

Let's Paint the Picture:
Protecting the Bump

When my wife was first pregnant, we lived in New York City and rode the subway twice a day, during rush hour, of course. Which meant no available seats, hurried passengers and overly shovey bystanders. We tried to take the early train in the morning and the later train after work - but that just led to us running across Broadway right in the middle of the busiest times.

I'd like to tell you about one Wednesday morning in particular. We had just made it to the platform in time to read the red blinking sign: *Next train 3 minutes.* I could feel everyone prepare to squeeze into the train by any means necessary.

My wife and I were the first people by the doors. As they opened, I put my arms around my wife's belly like an exaggerated belt made of steel. As we were walking in, a sweaty man in a suit elbowed us to get through.

Now, I don't know if you've seen any Jackie Chan movies. You know the ones where he's just super swift and fast to react? Does a little hip dip then an uppercut? Imagine that, but with less finesse and grace. That was me.

Why am I telling you this and why does it matter? Well, when your partner is pregnant you become overly defensive and protective. Your partner is no longer just your partner, she's your baby's mother. And that belly is the most precious thing you've ever seen.

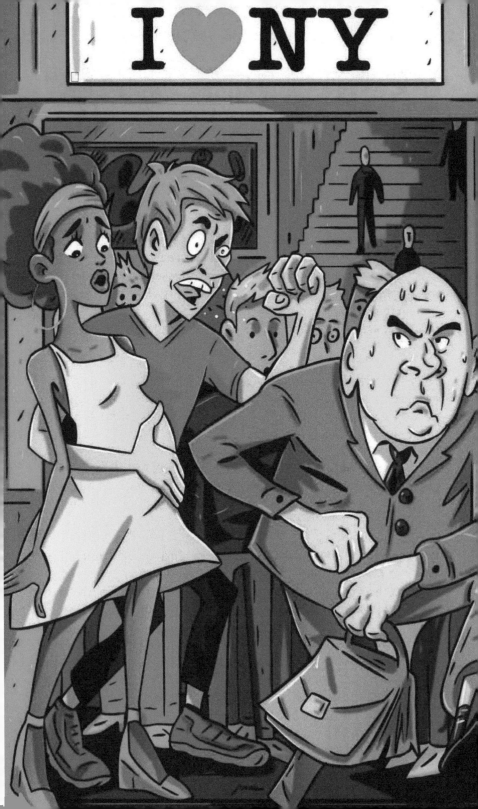

A short message from the Author:

Hey, are you enjoying our pregnancy guide?

We'd love to hear your thoughts!

Many readers do not realize how hard reviews are to come by

and how much they really help an author.

We would be incredibly grateful if you could take just 60 seconds to write a brief review on Amazon, even if it's just a few short lines!

Customer Reviews

⭐⭐⭐⭐⭐ 2
5.0 out of 5 stars ▾

5 star	▉▉▉▉▉	100%
4 star		0%
3 star		0%
2 star		0%
1 star		0%

See all verified purchase reviews ›

Share your thoughts with other customers

Write a customer review ⬅

Simply visit:

A m a z o n . c o m / R Y P

Your review will genuinely make a difference

and will help us gain exposure for our work.

Thank you in advance for taking the time to share your thoughts!

Welcome to Week 14
Babymoon Time:
Pack Those Bags, Baby!

_TL, DR_: *The second trimester is usually considered the easiest trimester for women due to a general decrease in pregnancy symptoms. Enjoy this time together with a babymoon!*

4 minute read

Fast facts covering:

- Joys of the Second Trimester
- Babymoon planning

They don't call the second trimester the "pregnancy honeymoon period" for nothing. Usually the most enjoyable time of pregnancy, as mom is generally feeling a lot better with an easing of her morning sickness, reduction in bathroom visits and potentially more energy.

Around this time is when couples decide to tackle the good old to-do list. Sure, there may be some lengthy things on there like setting up the nursery or picking out the proper car seat, but there is one super exciting one... planning the "babymoon!"

A "baby" what now?

Babymoon! A trip for mom and dad to get away before the baby arrives. This is a particularly special trip, though. It is usually pretty romantic but can also be adventurous (to a point). Stick with grounded activities and eat great food!

The main places to avoid is anywhere that has Zika. Within the US is generally considered safe and Zika free. Think beach resorts, gentle hiking areas, maybe a spa trip or perhaps even a staycation!?

It is important to remember the point of this trip is for both of you to fully relax and bask in each other's company.

If this is your first child, go all out! You won't have two other rug rats running around like my wife and I did when we were expecting our third. Eat late meals, lay on the beach and do things only a couple could do!

Week 14 Dad's Guide

Baby's Development

Size Estimate:
- Orange (get that Vitamin C up!)
- Wondering if your baby is happy or sad? They might not know either at this point, but there is bound to be some facial expressions forming around this week!
- There is a possibility your baby is sucking their thumb right this second!

Mom's Changes

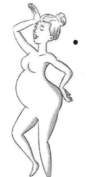

Physically:
New Symptoms:
- Teeth cleaning. This may sound a little strange to first-time dads, but around weeks 14-15 is the perfect time for mom to pay a visit to the dentist's office. Increased hormone levels can cause bacteria to build up leading to bleeding and swollen gums. This can progress to gingivitis which can actually

bring on early labor, putting your baby's health and safety at risk.

- "Round Ligament Pain" may arise around this time. It is caused by mom's uterus being stretched out to accommodate a growing baby, which may lead to stomach cramping.
- Ahhh, finally more sleep for mom with decreased nausea and fewer bathroom pit stops!
  Recurring Symptoms:
- Bloating and constipation.
  Emotionally:
- Most likely mom is filled with energy and excitement. She is also starting to feel like herself again!

Dad's Feelings

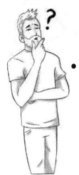

- With all this talk of the babymoon, you're most likely feeling anticipation for a romantic trip for two!

Supporting Mom

- That round ligament pain doesn't sound too pleasant. This week, you can help support mom by encouraging her to put her feet up and just get some rest. General resting and relaxation can help relieve her pains.
- Double-check that the 16 Week prenatal appointment is booked

Welcome to Week 15
Baby Budgeting:
Balancing Baby's Books

TL, DR: *Planning for upcoming costs including smart shopping tips and saving for baby's future*

5 minute read

Fast facts covering :

- Upcoming bills
- Cutting costs through savvy shopping!
- Savings ideas & options

There are many things you cannot control during pregnancy including mom's symptoms and baby's developments all the way up to when the actual labor begins. However, one thing you can plan for (barring unforeseen issues) is what upcoming expenses are associated with your baby's arrival.

Did You Know?	In the US, the average cost of a baby's first year is right around $13,000 (and that doesn't even include the cost of childbirth) Then, the expected cost to raise your child to age 17 totals an estimated $245,000. (*Source - USDA*)

Some examples of first-year costs include :

- Furniture, Baby Gear, Accessories (think: car seat, stroller, crib)
- Clothing
- Diapers, Wipes & Creams
- Health Insurance
- Food (to supplement breast milk or formula)

Second-hand Shopping!

There are a plethora of hand-me-down shops both online and in-person that offer baby goods at a fraction of the cost. The majority of these goods will be used, but as long as they are in good working condition, it could be a great alternative to purchasing new.

Also, expand your network to family and friends to see if there are any items they no longer need that would be beneficial to you. Mommy and daddy groups are also another great outlet for obtaining used baby items.

Pro Tip:	If you are planning to have more than one baby, then consider buying items that are unisex, for example colors and styles that would work for both boys and girls.

Saving for baby

Depending on what is important for you and your partner, there are a few routes you can go here. The two most popular being:

- **General savings account** at your local bank. You can set aside a fixed amount to contribute on a regular basis (EG. monthly) or decide to add money from special occasions and birthdays (or do both!)
- **529 Account** (*specifically for US readers*) is a more specialized option that is geared towards saving a certain amount of money that your child can use for educational purposes when they are of age. It is also possible for earnings to grow tax-free (at federal tax level).

Week 15 Dad's Guide

Baby's Development

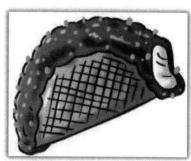

Size Estimate:

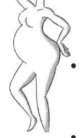

- Choco Taco (don't judge, they're a great late-night snack)
- Picture this - in the previous weeks, baby's eyes were located at the sides of baby's head and their ears were located around their neck! Now both eyes and ears are gradually moving into their rightful positions onto your baby's face … isn't that incredible!?
- Also, baby's bones and skeleton frame are now forming

Mom's Changes

Physically:
New Symptoms:

- Have you ever heard the old wives' tale that the more heartburn you have, the more hair your baby will have? Well, we won't know if that's true. But mom may experience heartburn around this week!
- The higher levels of blood flow circulating around mom's body can also cause nosebleeds to occur. Keep a lookout for this.

Recurring Symptoms:

- Frequent urination, bloating, constipation, and round ligament pain

Emotionally:

- Mom's most likely still feeling the relief of those first-trimester pregnancy symptoms. Enjoy it!

Dad's Feelings

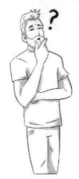

- With all this financial talk, you may be in a more familiar space and feeling a little more in control of things. This is a huge task ahead. So try to get planning ASAP to get on top of this early, as there are many more things coming up to prepare for!

Supporting Mom

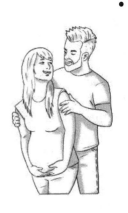

- If heartburn is affecting mom, it is sure to be uncomfortable for her. Not only does it affect her eating but it also can interfere with her sleep. The most helpful ways to support mom are:
  - Keeps snacks nearby which keep heartburn at bay (EG. nuts, crackers, non-citrus fruits, rice cakes, granola bars, caffeine-free herbal teas such as chamomile)
  - Have water handy at all times
  - Elevate pillows when mom is resting

Pro Tip:	What is mom's most dreaded household chore? Start doing it without her even asking you and she will absolutely love you for it!

Welcome to Week 16
16 Week Prenatal Appointment & Pregnancy Brain

**TL,DR**: 16-week prenatal appointment occurs, mom may experience some forgetfulness ("Pregnancy Brain") & baby can hear your voice!

4 minute read

Fast facts covering:

- Managing Pregnancy Brain
- 16 Week Prenatal

Forgetfulness during pregnancy is actually a real thing. It is experienced by some pregnant women and believed to be caused by multiple factors including lack of sleep, decreased energy levels and hormone changes. But don't worry, if your partner is affected by pregnancy brain, reassure them that it affects many pregnant women and that it's only a temporary condition which normally goes away within the first 10-12 weeks after birth.

Pro Tip:	Avoid misplacing everyday items by agreeing with your partner to leave them in a "common area" of the house. For example, leave house keys, car keys, purse, shoes, phone etc... in a specified location such as a hallway table or key bowl at the entrance of your home. Another idea is to buy her a small note pad or diary (if she doesn't currently have one), that she can carry around in her bag to write down important reminders, appointments and to-do lists or alternatively encourage her to use her cell phone's notes and calendar apps.

16 Week Prenatal Appointment - what can I expect?

Each prenatal usually includes a urine test and ultrasound (or doppler).

Whilst a baby's gender is normally detectable via ultrasound during weeks 18-20, although rare, you *may* be able to see it on this week's scan. (That is of course if you haven't already found out via NIPT blood testing mentioned in week 10).

Pro Tip:	Always try to come prepared with a few questions of your own (it also shows your partner that you care!). If no questions come to mind, turn the mic to your doctor. Ask them: "Doctor, is there anything else we need to know or plan for at this stage?"

Week 16 Dad's Guide

Baby's Development

Size Estimate:

- Light bulb (Q: How many Psychiatrists does it take to change a light bulb? A: Just one. But only if the light bulb really wants to change)
- Baby is sprouting little bones in their ears that allow them to hear you better! So don't be shy, keep talking and singing to them and get that baby bonding going right from the get-go!

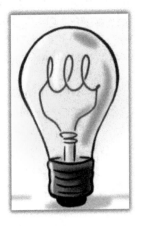

Pro Tip:	As baby can hear you, continue bonding by talking to them so they get used to your voice. If speaking directly to them feels strange, you can always just talk about your thoughts out aloud.

- Generally, around weeks 16-20 is when mom can feel baby's movements. They won't feel like heavy punches or kicks, but more like little butterflies flying around.

Mom's Changes

Physically:
New Symptoms:

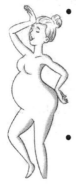

- It is commonly thought that women experience the best pregnancy symptom of all ... 'pregnancy glow'. This causes mom's skin to start glowing and she may also experience longer nails and thicker hair. Pregnancy glow is caused by higher levels of blood flowing around mom's body and those continuing hormonal changes.
- Though having that glow can be common for women, not everyone feels this way. Some women may experience self-esteem issues due to their weight gain.

Recurring Symptoms:
- Nosebleeds, round ligament pain, heartburn, and constipation

Emotionally:
- Mom may be feeling super confident right now thanks to that glow.
  - (Make sure you compliment her, a lot)
- If mom doesn't feel like she has the glow, make that girl glow!
  - (Make sure you compliment her, a lot)

Dad's Feelings

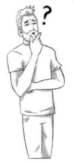

- You may be feeling some anticipation to soon be able to feel baby's kicks! Seeing mom filled with this new joy makes it feel all the more real.

Supporting Mom

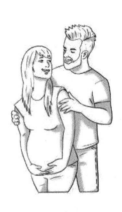

- A simple way to support mom this week is to listen to her explain what "quickening" feels like. This is a huge milestone that is personal to mom. At this stage, baby's movements are too minimal for others to feel and can normally only be felt by her.
- Show mom support as she may be a little self-conscious of her weight gain and increasingly growing belly! Remember to keep reminding her that a growing belly is a sign of a healthy pregnancy.
- Also ensure she's eating the right nutrient packed health foods as mentioned in previous weeks.

Pro Tip: As moms belly gets bigger, her spine begins bending which puts more strain on her back muscles and can cause back pains. Some ideas to help are: organizing a surprise prenatal massage for mom, give mom a back rub yourself or preparing a nice warm (not too hot!) bath (and even perhaps set the mood with some candles and dimmed lights). Other options are Yoga or Pilates.

Welcome to Week 17
Baby's Personal Bodyguard:
Bump Duty

TL,DR: *How to prepare for 'Tummy Touchers' and protecting that bump!*

3 minute read

Fast facts covering:

- Mom's precious baby bump

As mom's belly grows, you may experience two things:

1. Everyone (and their mother) wants to touch it

This can include family, friends, colleagues, and even strangers!

Some moms see it as a sign of affection and love it, whilst others can feel quite the opposite and be very protective, preferring a 'no-touch zone' approach. It's a good idea to check in with mom on her comfort levels and how she would like to deal with this situation when someone goes in for that next belly rub!

2. Some people don't notice it and can bump into the bump!

If the opposite is occurring and the bump is somehow 'invisible' to people and they're not giving it the space it deserves - create a human barrier! You know those bodyguards that protect celebs while they're out galivanting? Channel them.

Week 17 Dad's Guide

Baby's Development

Size Estimate:

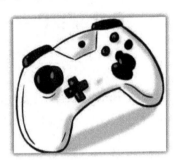

- Console Gaming Controller (recalling those late college nights)

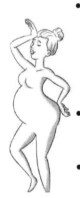

- The biggest change we're seeing from your baby this week is their skeleton changing from soft cartilage to bone. And on top of that bone? Some meat is starting to develop!
- Baby's umbilical cord is growing stronger and thicker by the day.

Mom's Changes

Physically:

New Symptoms:

- Odd behavior? Wondering why mom might be changing her underwear several times a day or taking multiple showers daily? This may be due to the increased bodily fluids that start around week 17.

Recurring Symptoms:

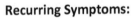

- Nosebleeds, round ligament pain, heartburn, and constipation

Emotionally:

- Mom could be feeling a bit disoriented due to the weird dreams she is having. This sounds familiar from week 8 when they were more anxiety-driven dreams. These are mainly caused by hormonal changes and perhaps a bit of lingering nervousness. They are known to be, well … a bit more out there…
- If she rolls over and gives you a funny smirk, just don't ask any questions. She has no feelings for her

high school boyfriend, these dreams are out of her control!

Dad's Feelings

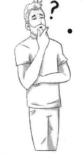

- You may be feeling like a true protector to your partner and baby. As the weeks roll by and the belly slowly grows, you may feel extra cautious and defensive about mom's baby bump when around other people (particularly out in public). Rest assured, it is totally normal to feel this way.

Supporting Mom

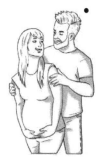

- Those wild dreams could be causing mom to lose some sleep. You can help support her by giving her some warm tea before bed or maybe purchase a relaxing light-hearted book for her to read before lights out. The more relaxed she is, the more likely she is to not only fall asleep but to stay asleep.

Pro Tip:	Dizziness is caused by an increased blood flow to baby and less to moms' brain. Mom needs to be careful with her growing bump as this can lead to unsteadiness and a higher chance of losing her balance. Ensure she is wearing flat comfortable shoes with grippy soles and possibly without laces for convenience during pregnancy, for example, running shoes. Perhaps a trip to the shops is in order! However, it's probably better to not surprise her since mom's feet can enlarge or swell during pregnancy, she may need to buy a half size larger to ensure she's comfortable. Also head to the shops towards the end of the day as this tends to be the time they swell up the most!

Month 4 Checklist & Reminders

(Because who has time to make their own list?)

☐   Start planning the babymoon

☐   Make a list of upcoming finances and savings plan options for baby

☐   Schedule the 20-week prenatal appointment and the anatomy screening

☐   Help mom navigate through pregnancy brain

☐   Protect that baby bump

MONTH 5 - Weeks 18 through 21
Learn about:

- **Gender Reveal:** *Party or surprise*

- **Dad mirroring Mom's Symptoms**: *Couvade syndrome*

- **Anatomy Screening**: *What to expect*

- **Naming Baby**: *bring on all the options!*

Let's Paint the Picture:
Revealing Baby's Gender

The car ride to Party City, which usually takes about fifteen minutes with no traffic, begins to feel like three and a half hours. I can't tell if it's the sheer excitement of what today will bring or the envelope burning a hole in my pocket.

I walk up to the balloon aisle standing behind an anxious mom gripping her son's hand as he screams how he wanted a red balloon, not a maroon balloon. The mom is trying to keep it together by telling him it is red, spoiler alert - he disagrees.

I zigzag past them to aisle three and cautiously slide over the envelope containing our baby's gender.

A twenty-something-year-old employee greets me with a smile and a nod. I watch her open it up and try to read if her eyes are telling me it's a boy or a girl. I'm pretty sure that was a "it's a boy" smile! No, wait, it was definitely a "daddy's little angel" smile.

After a five-minute wait, she hands me back a large balloon filled with the color signifying our baby's gender. I try to peek through the balloon for a pink or a blue. I think to myself, just two more hours until the reveal. Hold it together, dad.

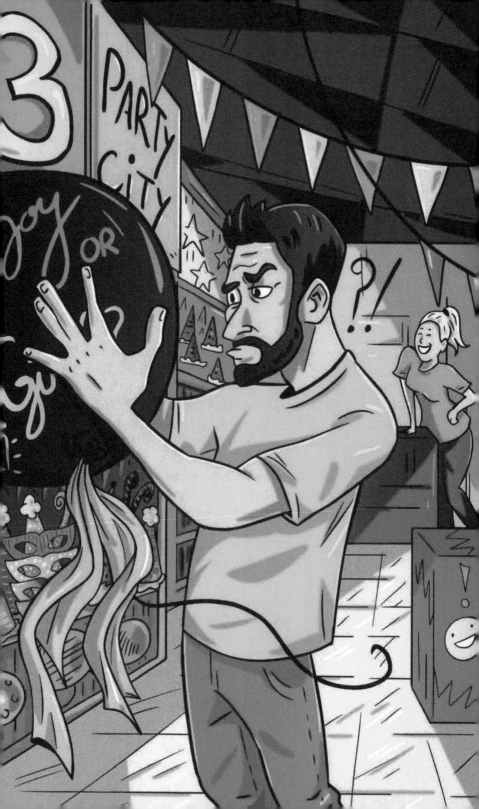

Welcome to Week 18
Baby's Gender:
Time For The Big Reveal

<u>TL, DR</u>: *Learning baby's gender & deciding whether to reveal privately or throw a gender reveal party*

4 minute read

Fast facts covering:

- Planning for Baby's Gender Reveal

Baby's gender may already be known by now if you opted for the genetic blood testing (or NIPT as discussed in week 10). Otherwise, if you decide to wait, then between weeks 18 and 20, the Anatomy screening will take place revealing your baby's gender. We'll dive into this a bit more in Week 20, but for this week let's focus on one key piece of information you will have access to baby's sex!

You should have an open conversation with your partner prior to the screening to determine if you want to find out then or wait. This will be one of the first questions the ultrasound technician will ask you.

Throw a Party?

A very popular option is to throw a gender reveal party with friends and family to announce your baby's sex. The couple finds out at this time as well. The doctor's office will provide your baby's sex to you, usually in an envelope. Once this is obtained, there are many ways to plan the announcement, but a couple of popular ones are:

- **Gender reveal cake!** Give the envelope to a bakery and ask them to make a cake with a certain color filling inside to signify a girl or boy. EG. blue for boy and pink for a girl. Cut the cake open at the party!

- **Balloon Pop!** Have a store fill up a balloon with the confetti of the "color of the sex". Pop the balloon to find out!

Or reveal it privately?

If you would prefer a more private reveal just for the two of you, the possibilities are endless! Some options are:

- Plan a special dinner for two where you reveal over dessert!
- Go for a scenic hike and open the envelope when you get to the top of your destination!

Otherwise, if you've got the patience and the willpower, waiting till birth can be an amazing surprise. You can think of this as your own private gender reveal party that you and your partner can experience together once your baby is born!

We found out the sex for two of our three children early on, but honestly - finding out on delivery day was one of the best surprises you will ever experience!

Pro Tip:	There're so many ideas and different ways to reveal your baby's gender. See for yourself - do a quick Google or YouTube search "Gender Reveal Ideas" and if deciding to throw a party, start thinking about invitations!

Week 18 Dad's Guide

Baby's Development

Size Estimate:

- Pint of Ben and Jerrys
- Your baby may have learned how to hiccup by now, which mom can

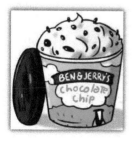

possibly start feeling as small movements in her belly.

- Things to look out for in your next ultrasound:
    - Baby's genitals are starting to form and can possibly be seen (more so for boys).
    - Also, your baby may have learned how to yawn, so keep your eyes peeled!

Mom's Changes

Physically:

New Symptoms:

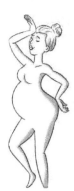

- Normally moms begin to feel their first 'major' baby movements anywhere from now to week 22. This can vary depending on mom's height, weight, body type, and baby's positioning in the womb. Mom may think she's experiencing gas or an upset stomach but in fact, this could actually be baby moving!
- Increased appetite. Mom may be feeling pretty ravenous! Remind her to eat slow and sit up after eating to keep the discomfort away such as heartburn.
- Mom may experience dizziness caused by less blood flow to her and more to baby, so advise her to stand up slowly when in a seated position.
- Some other symptoms mom may be feeling are backaches, swelling in hands and feet, and trouble sleeping.

Emotionally:

- Deciding if you want to find out the sex of your baby can be overwhelming. At week 18, mom has about two weeks to make this decision. The good thing is, while mom may be feeling the pressure, you can both decide to not find out for the time being and can always inquire about baby's gender at a later date when you are ready.

Dad's Feelings

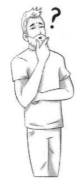

- You may be feeling excited about the upcoming week 20 anatomy screening and possible gender reveal. You finally get an up-close at your baby!

Supporting Mom

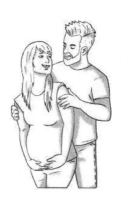

- Week 18 is a busy one! You have the anatomy screening coming up and mom has a few new symptoms she is feeling. Try to carve some time for a date night!
- Advise mom that it's important she sleeps on her side (ideally left side). Not only is it generally the most comfortable position for pregnant moms but is also recognized as the safest position for baby's safety from now up until childbirth. It ensures less pressure on mom's internal organs such as her intestines, and therefore doesn't restrict nutrients from passing to baby.
- Double-check that the 20 Week prenatal appointment is booked

Pro Tip:	If mom experiences swelling of hands and feet, it may feel like "pins and needles". If this happens, recommend mom to regularly perform hand, wrist, ankle and feet stretches to relieve those tingling sensations. Also putting her feet up as much as she can, taking regular walks and drinking lots of water can alleviate any discomforts.

Welcome to Week 19
Dad Experiencing Mom's Symptoms?
Couvade Syndrome

<u>TL, DR</u>: *Dad may have similar pregnancy symptoms as mom & mom may start to experience leg cramping.*

3 minute read

Fast facts covering:

- Couvade Syndrome (or Sympathetic Pregnancy)

Could it be true? Can Dad really be feeling similar symptoms as Mom? Not to hit you all with this incredibly technical-sounding term, but this is formally known as 'Couvade Syndrome' (also called Sympathetic Pregnancy).

So, what does it mean? Although this condition is not officially medically recognized, sometimes men can start to gain weight, feel nauseous, experience backaches and cramping, and follow along with other pregnancy symptoms simultaneously with mom each week. There are many people who disagree with this and say it is impossible - but on the other hand, there have also been many cases proving that it does exist!

"Couvade" is originally a French term which means to brood, which in pregnancy terms, 'loosely' translates to mean "we're pregnant". (Pronounced *"koo-vahd"*.)

MONTH 6 - Weeks 22 through 27
Learn about:

+ **Creating a Baby Registry**: *Consider must-haves and nice to haves*

+ **Making a Birth Plan**: *including your involvement*

+ **Baby Shower**: *time to party and let loose*

+ **Prep for Glucose Test**: *by supporting mom before and after*

+ **Tour Hospital**: *equipped with questions to ask*

+ **Childbirth Classes**: *throw on that thinking cap*

Let's Paint the Picture:
Creating Baby Registry

Just last night we snuggled in bed while I rubbed my wife's belly. Our pillow talk consisted of diaper brands, car seat adapters, and wipe warmers. Prior to pregnancy, our talks before bed were minimal, and our activity was spontaneous. Those days are in the past for a while. We work on the number 1 plan for this week...

Mission: "Figure Out Registry" - Underway!

Fast forward to this morning, we're in the middle of BuyBuyBaby. We circle around the store three times with one of those price-checking guns. As we aim and click, we see the items appear as a digitized list on the side of the gun.

We get sidetracked and caught up in a hushed but heated debate on why it matters that my mother suggested we purchase a bottle warmer. I tell her, well she raised six of us, and we turned out fine. Surely, the bottle warmer isn't going to harm our baby. She replies back that while these facts were true, they were dated. As I hold the bottle warmer with two thoughts in my head: 1. Fight for the bottle warmer and stand my ground 2. Let this slide and tell her that although she is not always right, she is *never wrong*. I go with option 2 which was definitely the right choice as she squeezes my arm and tells me I'm the best husband in the world. I make a mental note to bring this up when our baby doesn't want to drink cold milk at 1am and would prefer a nice warm bottle.

By the end of the day we have 75 items on our registry: 50 must-haves, 20 nice-to -haves, and 5 that serve little to no purpose but are "cute!"

I've never spent so much time in a store and left without a single purchased item. Now, we wait for the baby shower!

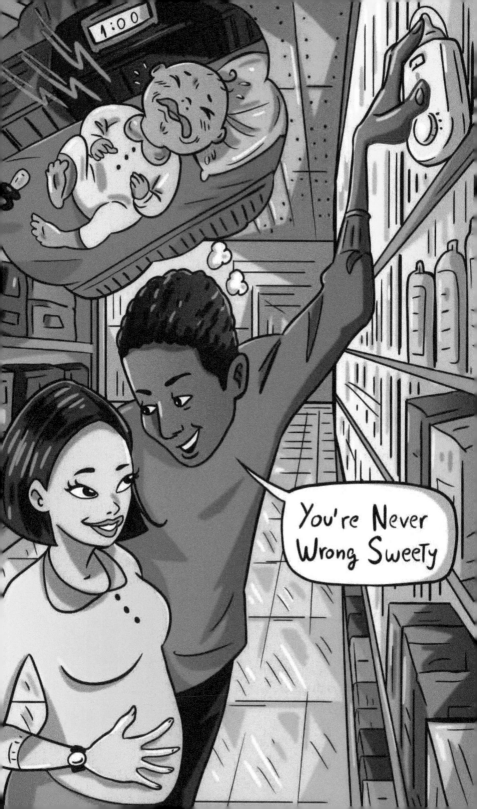

Welcome to Week 22
Baby Registry:
Diapers & Gadgets Galore

TL,DR: *Getting started on a baby registry.*

5 minute read

Fast facts covering:

- Creating your baby registry

Maybe you're married and made a wedding registry. Maybe this is your first-time cruising around the store with one of those fun price guns. Or maybe you can't be bothered to go to the store so you're sitting comfortably at home clicking each item.

Whatever your method is, this is usually a somewhat lengthy process that may involve some healthy arguing. The best way to approach this is to go in with a plan. Talk to some of your seasoned friends and family that have had kids and see what items they found useful and recommend. Compare and contrast different brands of items for the highest rated products. Then determine with your partner what is important for you both. Here are some items to kick you off, which in my opinion, are *must-haves*: car seat, stroller, crib, diapers and wipes, bathing tub, first aid kit, high chair, clothing, bottles. *Nice-to-haves*: Baby carrier, wipe warmer and wipe holder, diaper pail, sound machine, nursing pillows, light blocking blinds.

Big or small ticket items?

I would suggest adding a variety of lower-priced and higher-priced items. This allows the people who have access to your registry to buy the baby products that are within their budget and comfort zone.

What sizes?

For diapers and clothes, you will quickly see how fast a baby can grow. One day they are wearing a baggy newborn diaper, and two weeks later they may be the next size up! The same may be true for clothing. Make sure you put them in your favorite outfits soon and often to get use out of them. The best rule of thumb is to request clothing and diaper sizes that range from newborn to toddler.

Week 22 Dad's Guide

Baby's Development

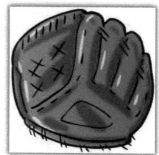

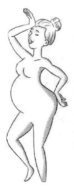

Size Estimate:
- Baseball Mitt (picture yourself on the front lawn practicing with your kid!)
- Your baby may have reached a new milestone of weighing a pound!
- Baby will start using their hands to try and grab objects within their reach such as their umbilical cord and nose.

Mom's Changes

Physically:
New Symptoms:
- Thanks to mom's hormone changes and the extra oil her body is producing, this can trigger an acne outbreak.
- With a growing belly, may come some new back pain and trouble catching her breath.
Recurring Symptoms:
- Stretch marks, heartburn, swollen hands and feet, constipation, and leg cramps.

Emotionally:

- While mom still has some time until labor, she may start feeling some fear. No matter how well she may prepare herself, it is a different world once labor actually begins. It is important to stay calm and do research to stay educated on different scenarios. So keep reading…!

Dad's Feelings

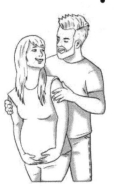

- If that registry is going well, you may be feeling pretty relieved and accomplished! If it's not, you might be feeling the pressure. If it is the latter, just remember - keep gift receipts and feel free to exchange items you didn't end up needing for items you do need.

Supporting Mom

- In mom's downtime, she may be overthinking some aspects of pregnancy or labor. From my own experience, I would suggest actively listening to your partner with a totally unbiased opinion. Keep in mind that she will be the one to go through the actual labor and experience pregnancy firsthand. It certainly doesn't hurt to reassure her that things will be OK, but if she is panicking that labor will be incredibly intense (it probably will), just listen, respect her feelings and be a sounding board for her.
- Double-check that the 24 Week prenatal appointment is booked

Did You Know? Did you know that approximately 80% of females experience sleeping difficulties whilst pregnant? You can help mom by ensuring she's side sleeping (on her left to avoid putting pressure on vital blood vessels) and perhaps using that pregnancy pillow we mentioned to maximize her comfort as much as possible.

Welcome to Week 23
Birth Plans: *The Best Laid Plans...*

TL, DR: *Start Birth Plan discussions with mom and why your involvement is so important.*

5 minute read

Fast facts covering:

- What is a Birth Plan?
- The important role you play

At 23 weeks, it may seem a bit premature to make a birth plan. However, they are normally shared with the doctor or midwife anywhere from weeks 30-35. These are huge decisions that are best decided on carefully and without haste.

A birth plan outlines mom's wishes before, during and after labor and normally includes things such as :

- *Who* she would like to be present at each stage?
- *How* she would like her body positioned during labor
- *Whether* she would like coaching on how and when to push
- *Who* cuts the umbilical cord and what happens with the placenta?
- *What* happens with your baby immediately after delivery, e.g. baby dried off, skin to skin, feed your baby...?
- *What* she would like to do with baby's cord blood
- Pain relief preferences

> **Note:** You can find many examples of birth plans online. Simply search for "Birth Plan Templates".

It is also important to remember that the birth plan may not always go accordingly due to unforeseen events. As the saying goes, even "the best-laid plans often go awry", which can be especially true for childbirth.

Your Involvement

During labor, moms discover the important role dads play and how much they assist in the labor process as their birthing partner. This highlights the importance of why you need to be involved in the birth plan right from the get-go!

Some things you may wish to consider:

- Are you comfortable cutting the cord?
- Do you want to have skin to skin contact with your baby straight after mom?
- If your baby is experiencing difficulties being delivered, are you comfortable with the use of forceps or a vacuum to guide your baby out?
- If mom has complications or is unable to leave the bed, will you accompany your baby during any tests?
- How much does mom want to be photographed or filmed before, during and after?

Week 23 Dad's Guide

Baby's Development

Size Estimate:

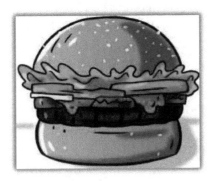

- Whopper Burger (Have It Your Way - while you still can!)
- As baby's kicks and punches

grow stronger, you may be able to start seeing them from the outside of mom's belly!

- Around week 23, your baby starts experiencing a more rapid increase in weight and may double from approximately one to two pounds over the next month. Remember, if mom is feeling down about her weight, remind her it's a sign of a healthy baby!

Mom's Changes

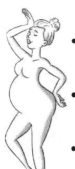

Physically:
New Symptoms:

- Mom can expect to start feeling even more movement from baby!

Recurring Symptoms:

- Backaches, stretch marks and itchy skin, heartburn, swollen hands and feet, and leg cramps.

Emotionally:

- Mom may be feeling really excited about the new movements from your baby. It is the perfect distraction from some of the more uncomfortable symptoms.

Dad's Feelings

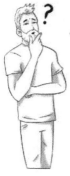

- Being fully involved in creating a co-birth plan may help you feel empowered! You will be the closest person in the room to your partner, so your support is incredibly important and necessary during labor and delivery. Continue staying involved and discuss the topics on mom's birth plan together!

Supporting Mom

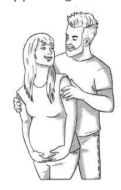

- Lean over and reach for that belly! You may be surprised to see how much this means to mom. Now that baby's kicks are more powerful and you can probably feel them - this is an experience you and mom can share. Take some video footage as a precious memory to look back on and to show your child when they are older!

Discussion Point:	**Birth Doula** - Speak with your partner on whether she wants to use a 'birth doula'. They are basically a person trained in childbirth that provide emotional and physical support to mom during labor and delivery. They assist mom with breathing and pain relief techniques during labor and some women find that they don't require as much pain medication (if any at all) with a birth doula's guidance. On the other hand, you might be all the support that she needs!

Pro Tip:	If Braxton Hicks contractions are bothering mom, help her get more comfortable by ensuring she's staying well hydrated with water and regularly switching positions.

Welcome to Week 24
Baby Shower Planning: *Let's Party!*

TL, DR: *Preparing for your baby shower that generally occurs between 28-33 weeks.*

4 minute read

Fast facts covering:

- What's in a Baby Shower?
- Are you (and other male friends) invited?

First off, happy six months of pregnancy! Time really does fly when you're creating life.

If you and mom decide on having a baby shower to celebrate your baby, this is usually held between 28-33 weeks, so planning should start soon. It is usually organized by family and/or friends and it may include receiving baby shower gifts and playing fun games such as gender guessing, sometimes before an actual gender is revealed at the party itself. However, this is entirely up to you and your partner, so make sure to share your thoughts of what you would like!

In terms of location, this can also vary depending on preference. It can be held outdoors, in a venue, a family member's home, and anywhere in between. (Vote for indoors with the air on if it's during the summer months)

Remember, this occasion is a great time for mom, as she is able to let loose and celebrate the homecoming of your little one.

Pro Tip:	Organize with party hosts to hold a "diaper raffle" with baby shower guests. This is a great way to collect diapers of all sizes while providing the guests with a fun gift too!

A typical diaper raffle will involve giving each person a ticket for the number of diapers they give. The tickets will be randomly selected and the winner(s) receive a small prize, usually a picture frame, spa gift, or candles.

Can we play too?

Back in the day, this was usually a big no-no, but with the times changing, this has taken a turn as well. It is now pretty normal for a dad and even other men to be at the shower. Having said that, perhaps something you should discuss with your partner before inviting the whole crew!

On the other hand, if you would rather sit this out, then it is still totally acceptable to either drop your partner off at the shower or pick her up. If the shower will be at your home, you can greet guests and/or join your wife to say goodbye. This way, you are able to make an appearance while supporting your wife, without committing to the entire shower.

Week 24 Dad's Guide

Baby's Development

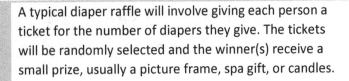

Size Estimate:

- Full 12 Inch Sub (there we go, you finally get the full sub)
- Baby's face is now close to being fully developed, so you may get a glimpse of what they look like at your next scan!

- Interestingly, baby's hair growing on their face and head is completely white, as a result of not yet having any color pigmentation!

Mom's Changes

Physically:

New Symptoms:

- Pregnancy swelling can lead to Carpal Tunnel Syndrome. Mom may experience a tingling or numbness in her wrists or hands so be sure to recommend regular hand stretching exercises and perhaps even trying a wrist brace. Don't worry, it is another common symptom affecting over 50% of all pregnant women.

Recurring Symptoms:

- Backaches, Braxton Hicks, stretch marks, heartburn, swollen hands and feet, constipation, and leg cramps.

Emotionally:

- There can be a lot of pressure in making sure mom is eating healthy, exercising, and being careful in daily activities. As a result, from time to time, mom may experience feelings of anxiety about her own and baby's health. Therefore, it's important that you encourage open conversations about both of your emotional states and to remember that much of what you're both feeling is totally normal.

Heads Up:	Mom may experience temporary slight blurred vision due to her hormone levels causing a change in her tear production. If she has this, don't worry too much as it normally doesn't last and more often than not disappears after birth. During this time, mom may feel more comfortable wearing glasses rather than contact lenses. If she suspects something more than just blurred vision, you should consult her eye specialist.

Dad's Feelings

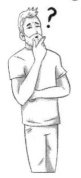

- Registry: check, Baby Shower Discussion: check. You're most likely feeling pretty accomplished right now! There are still quite a few things to do before baby, but hey, we checked off a couple of important items!

Supporting Mom

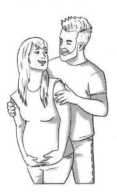

- Ahh, that carpal tunnel I mentioned. This can be incredibly uncomfortable for mom. Some ideas for you to help her are: gently massaging her wrists and encouraging her to elevate her wrists while in use. For example when typing on keyboard.
- Double-check that mom's Glucose Appointment is booked, as it is normally scheduled for any time over the next 4 weeks (we cover this next week).

Did You Know? Before the end of Trimester 2 (week 27) mom's breasts will be fully prepared for breast feeding just in case baby arrives ahead of schedule! And her breasts may even start leaking milk! This early form of milk is known as 'Colostrum'. On that note, it may be an opportune time to start having discussions with mom on whether she would prefer to breast or bottle feed and what role she would like you to play. For example, she may want to breastfeed during the day and then by night, she may want you to take over with bottle feeding duties.

Welcome to Week 25
Glucose Test: *Sip, Sip, Mom*

TL, DR: *Helping mom prepare & supporting her for glucose screening. This tests if she has the temporary pregnancy condition "gestational diabetes".*

3 minute read

Fast facts covering:

- What is a glucose test?
- How you can help & support

Your first thought maybe, my partner doesn't have diabetes so why the need for the test? Great question! The keyword here is gestational, which basically means during pregnancy. Gestational diabetes is a very common pregnancy condition that normally goes away after birth. The gestational diabetes screening checks mom's glucose levels during pregnancy.

The test is super simple and consists of:

1. Mom drinks a sugar-filled liquid over an hour-long period. (Note: it isn't the tastiest drink and can sometimes cause a pretty nasty headache.)
2. After the hour, her blood work is drawn to see how her body processed the sugar.
3. It can then take up to a week to get the result back.

How can you be of service?

The best way to be of service is to accompany mom to the appointment and be sure to have a snack on-hand for after the test. Once done, keep mom occupied and her mind off the testing until the results are back.

Note: Don't panic if she has an abnormal result. She will just have to take a more in-depth test, potentially make some dietary adjustments and be monitored a little more closely. If so, she will need your support to stay on track!

Week 25 Dad's Guide

Baby's Development

Size Estimate:

- Size 12 Shoe (You know what they say about big feet? Big socks!)
- "You spin me right round, baby right round!" Baby has now developed a sense of direction and can now determine which way is up and down.
- Baby's nose is now developed and functioning and can start smelling scents in the womb.

Fun Fact: If you are having a boy, his testicles begin to drop into his scrotum area, a journey which can take up to 3 long months!

Mom's Changes

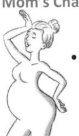

Physically:
New Symptoms:

- One thing to distract mom from her potentially growing feet is a new symptom called - hemorrhoids. Hemorrhoids occur when the baby puts too much pressure on mom's digestive tract.

These swollen anal veins can be very painful, itchy, and uncomfortable. They make it difficult to use the bathroom or even sit down.

- Restless leg syndrome (or RLS). This one might be hard for mom to explain to you, but it is basically a sensation that is felt in mom's legs when she is laying down or relaxing. It is almost like a constant urge to have to move. It can be very disruptive so make sure to sympathize with mom a little extra on this one.

Important:	If mom notices that her skin is more pale and lighter colored than usual, this could be an early sign of anemia and low iron levels. Although this is very common during pregnancy, get it checked out by your doctor.

Recurring Symptoms:

- Backaches, Braxton Hicks, stretch marks, heartburn, swollen hands and feet, trouble sleeping, frequent urination and leg cramps. On the bright side, mom's energy levels may still be quite good.

Did You Know?	During pregnancy, moms can experience an increase in shoe size and unlike many of the other pregnancy symptoms, this one may last even after pregnancy!

Emotionally:

- If mom took her glucose test this week, she may be anxiously awaiting the results. It is important to remember that half of pregnancy is waiting for results or your baby to come, so now is a great time to practice the fun art of patience.

Dad's Feelings

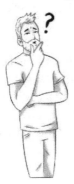

- You, understandably, maybe feeling a bit left out. Mom is experiencing everything firsthand. She may have less time for you than she normally does, as she is navigating through life with a child growing inside of her. Instead of expressing these feelings which may result in her feeling bad, just try to spend more time together doing some of your old favorite activities. Maybe don't go rock climbing, but do go to a movie or have a picnic in the sunshine!

Supporting Mom

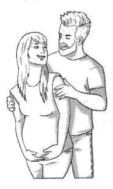

- If mom's experiencing hemorrhoids, ensure she is drinking enough water and eating a high fiber diet which will help her stools to pass more easily. Also, help mom relieve the pain by applying a cool pack to the affected area.
- Support mom by going on a shoe shopping trip. What's better than fitting in your old shoes? Buying a ton of new ones...

Did You Know?	Since your baby's listening skills are progressing each week, if they hear sounds and songs regularly, these same sounds and songs can make them feel comfortable and relaxed after birth. Start speaking and playing your favorite songs to them now!

Welcome to Week 26
Touring The Hospital:
Scope out the New Digs

TL, DR: *Birthplace options & touring the hospital prior to delivery to familiarize yourselves.*

Important Note:	For the sake of this book, we will focus on hospital births since 98-99% of women deliver at a hospital compared to a home birth or birthing center. Additionally, if you take the tour this week, you may be able to take childbirth classes at the same time! If you go this route, be sure to also check out week 27 to learn all about childbirth classes.

5 minute read

Fast facts covering:

- Considering where to give birth
- Touring labor and delivery hospital
- Important questions to ask

There are a few options for places to deliver. You have your hospitals, birth centers, or home births. It usually comes down to two things when determining which to choose.

First, if your doctor advises that mom's pregnancy is high risk or you are pregnant with twins or mom has had a prior c section - then nine times out of ten, the delivery would be at a hospital.

Secondly, if your partner feels they would need or want any medical interventions in the form of pain relief such as Epidural, Pethidine or Nitrous Oxide (*refer to Glossary*) then again, a hospital is the way to go.

In addition to the above two main factors, here is a quick summary of them all:

- Hospital
  - Pro - complete medical supplies and resources
  - Con - may be pushed into an induction or c section if labor is not progressing fast enough
- Birthing Center
  - Pros - more holistic, typically able to labor as long as needed, more "homely" than hospitals, no medical interventions, average cost is a lot less than hospitals
  - Con - if things go awry mom will need to be sent to the hospital anyway for assistance
- Home Births
  - Pros - very similar to the birthing center and you are in a familiar and comfortable setting at home
  - Cons - again, similar to the birthing center con but also insurance may not cover any accrued charges

Hospital Tour Time!

The hospital where your baby will be delivered depends on which one is affiliated with your doctor's office. Each office (doctor or midwives) has at least one hospital that they have rights to. Once you are made aware of this, it's time to tour the hospital!

You can usually find the tour dates on the hospital website, or by simply calling in. Schedule a tour for you and your partner and come prepared with important questions to ask! (*Reminder to also ask about childbirth classes*).

> **Pro Tip:** Take note of where you can park, if you need a ticket, general layout of the hospital, visiting hours, and where the entrance is for the maternity ward. Also, ask for the paperwork to preregister for mom's delivery as it will save you valuable time on labor day.

Important Questions to Ask

This can get a bit lengthy, but I have narrowed down to the most crucial ones:

- What is the Nicu level?
    - 4 is the highest. If it's low, then they may have to transfer baby if extra help is needed.
- C Section policy and rate?
    - Can you be in the room with your partner the entire time?
    - Is skin to skin done right away? Is it only with mom or you too?
    - How many c-sections are performed each year?
- Baby-friendly?
    - Are all tests done bedside as opposed to baby leaving the room?
- Policy for you staying the night.
    - Is there a bed for you and is complimentary food included?
- Visiting hours
    - When can friends and family come see the baby, and when can't they?

Week 26 Dad's Guide

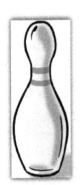

Baby's Development
Size Estimate:

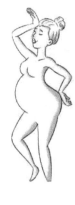

- **Bowling Pin** (Split Happens!)
- Baby is really starting to prepare for life on the outside, as their eyes will now start to open and they have also been practicing how to swallow and breathe. However, no air is currently being swallowed, still only amniotic fluid!

Fun Fact:	The flashlight test! If you take a flashlight to mom's belly, your baby may be able to notice the light and might start moving around!

Mom's Changes
Physically:
New Symptoms:

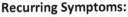

- Welcome: Insomnia! Mom may be struggling to sleep due to ongoing physical symptoms keeping her up and any anxious thoughts she may be having.

Recurring Symptoms:
- Backaches, Braxton Hicks, stretch marks, heartburn, swollen hands and feet, trouble sleeping, pregnancy brain, hemorrhoids, and leg cramps.

Emotionally:
- If mom toured the hospital this week, reality has probably set in big time. She saw the bed, the delivery room, and met some of the nurses. Just being in the hospital is enough to throw some moms into a whirlwind. On the other hand, mom

may be feeling way more relaxed now that she has familiarized herself with it all.

Dad's Feelings

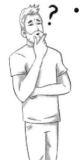

- Making it to the hospital on time during labor might feel like a scene straight out of 2 Fast 2 Furious. Hopefully, you are also feeling more relaxed after taking the practice drive there for the tour. If you are feeling overwhelmed, look back on the questions and answers from your tour and finalize any remaining uncertainties you may have.

Supporting Mom

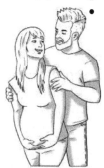

- With the possible onset of insomnia, she is most likely feeling exhausted with little to no energy throughout the day. Keep mom as relaxed as possible and encourage daytime napping. Also, it would certainly help to take any chores off of her hands and add them to your to-do list.

Pro Tip:	If mom is struggling to sleep at night, ensure she is getting enough exercise during the day and breathing in plenty of fresh air. Also suggest not to drink anything too close before bed as it can be difficult to get back to sleep after frequent bathroom visits!

Welcome to Week 27
Childbirth Classes:
Sharpen That pencil, Dad!

__TL, DR__: *Start scheduling childbirth classes to educate yourself & mom on labor, pain relief, nursing, and infant CPR.*

3 minute read

Fast facts covering:

- Childbirth classes
- Other useful classes to consider

As mentioned in week 26, you may wish to schedule your childbirth classes on the same day as your hospital tour for convenience, since the classes are normally held on-site. Alternatively, there are other options such as attending a local instructor's class or virtual online webinars. Booking is easy and can be made online and if you have insurance, ask them if they cover the costs. The instructor will most likely be a nurse or doctor, so come prepared with your questions as they will certainly have the best answers for you.

Be proactive, take the initiative, and start looking into these classes asap, as some do have waiting lists and you don't want to leave it too close to mom's due date. Take action now!

Recommended Topics

There will most likely be a wide array of classes offered, so sign up for as many as you find useful. Some suggestions are:

- Childbirth 101
- Coping with Pain
- Breastfeeding 101
- Infant CPR

Week 27 Dad's Guide

Baby's Development

Size Estimate:

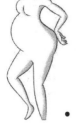

- Apple Pie ("This one time, at Childbirth class ...")
- Even though baby has been listening to you and mom for a while now and already recognises your voices, their hearing is somewhat muffled as their ears are still covered in that Vernix Caseosa we spoke about in week 19.

Fun Fact:	Around week 27 is when you may be able to start hearing baby's heartbeat through mom's belly. Gently press your ear to various spots of mom's tummy to see if you can hear it!

Mom's Changes

Physically:
New Symptoms

- Snissing! I wish this was as fun as it sounded, but it is simply peeing a little (or a lot) when you sneeze. It is caused by baby applying extra pressure on mom's bladder and this lovely symptom is likely to stick around after pregnancy as well. *(note: although not a real word, it's commonly referenced during pregnancy).*

Recurring Symptoms:

- Backaches, Braxton Hicks, RLS, stretch marks, heartburn, hemorrhoids, swollen hands and feet, trouble sleeping, constipation and leg cramps

Emotionally:

- All that childbirth talk might have mom feeling apprehensive about labor. One of the biggest things a lot of parents feel after the class is that real labor is nothing like the movies. Which can either be comforting or alarming.

Dad's Feelings

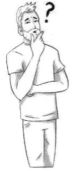

- You may have had some sleepless nights thinking about what to expect during childbirth. It feels so far away, but that due date is quickly approaching. After taking childbirth classes, you can hopefully get a bit more shut-eye from filling in any educational gaps you had prior. This is the best way you can prepare for the unknown of childbirth!

Supporting Mom

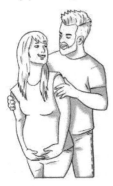

- Debrief with mom on how she feels after the childbirth classes. Reassure her that, although she will be the one going through the pain, you will be there every step of the way. Ask her what she would like you to do before, during and after labor. Make a list for yourself, and tackle these as the date approaches.
- Double-check that the 28-week prenatal appointment is booked.

Pro Tip:	As we enter the third trimester (next week), get ready to attend a lot more prenatal appointments. They will start occurring every 2 weeks and then soon move to weekly.

Month 6 Checklist & Reminders
(Because who has time to make their own list?)

☐   Finalize that baby registry!

☐   Start working on the birth plan

☐   Get excited for the upcoming baby shower!

☐   Support mom during Glucose Testing

☐   Scope out the labor and delivery hospital

    ☐   While there, pre-register

☐   Schedule Childbirth classes

☐   Schedule 28-week prenatal appointment

Part 3 - Third Trimester: The Final Countdown!
(Includes Weeks 28 through 42)

MONTH 7 - Weeks 28 through 31
Learn about:

- **Schedule Maternity Photoshoot:** *glam time, mom*

- **Look into a Push Present:** *spoil your partner a bit*

- **Finding a Pediatrician:** *interviewing your baby's doctor*

- **Childcare Options:** *the best choice for your family and wallet*

- **Parental Leave:** *make it easy to leave and return after*

Let's Paint the Picture:
The Search for Childcare

T rusting someone to watch your child is like the adult version of a trust fall. Except instead of worrying about falling, you're filled with anxiety about failing your child at the hands of someone else.

Which brings me to my current situation. My wife and I are huddled around the kitchen table with various pieces of paper, crossed out names, and markers of assorted colors. If I didn't know any better, I'd think it was a scene from Stranger Things.

Except we're not trying to find the Demogorgon or save Will. We're trying to find a babysitter who can provide our kid with the same support we would. Yet, as the saying goes, no one will love your child as much as you do.

Nevertheless, we must venture on and tackle this list with open eyes and a careful view...

First on the list - my mother. I added that name last night after my wife had gone to bed. I did my best to mirror her handwriting in hopes that her lack of sleep would blur her to this small addition.

She glances over it and moves to the next name. "Phew", I think. I'm in the clear. She didn't cross it out or question it. Maybe there is hope for dear old mom.
I mean, I turned out fine, right?

We end up asking my mother to come to help out. A "trial run" as my wife calls it. The list we provide to her is excessive, to say the least. We have appointed bathroom breaks... for my mother, not

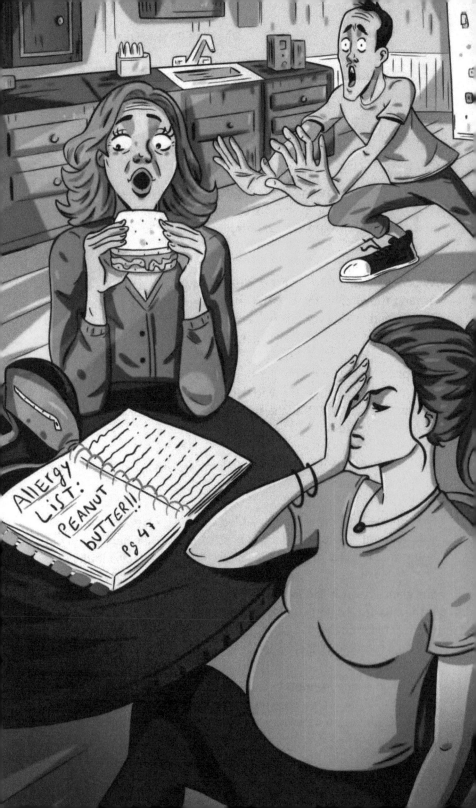

our child. But that's not the icing on the cake, the true peak of paranoia occurs when my mother pulls out her peanut butter sandwich. It looks innocent. No harm there. The corners are cut and the jelly was applied with just enough of a slight spillover.

My wife slides over the checkered binder sectioned off by category and abruptly flips to page forty-seven. Clear as day, it states:

Allergy List: (foods to avoid)
- *Peanut butter*

I wonder if my mom has lost the job at that moment. If only she had made a jelly jelly sandwich.

My wife and mother burst out laughing at the ridiculous nature of our binder. My mom eats the sandwich while my wife rubs her pregnant belly. They spend the rest of the afternoon discussing baby names, and out comes another list.

Welcome to Week 28
Surprise & Spoil Mom:
C'mon, She Deserves It!

<u>TL,DR</u>: *Dedicate this week to making mom feel special with a maternity photoshoot (you can join in, too!) and purchase a push present for her.*

3 minute read

Fast facts covering:

- Maternity Photoshoot!
- Push present
- 28 Week Prenatal Appointment

We can't move much further without acknowledging what week 28 begins... the third trimester! Ahh, remember your little embryo? Just look at them now!

Maternity Photoshoot

Week 28 is the perfect time to schedule a maternity photoshoot for mom. The bump is just big enough to show, and mom's trimester two energy levels are hopefully still around! Once the third trimester really ramps up, so does her added discomfort, so let's get these pictures in now.

Maternity photos can be shared with loved ones as everyone awaits your baby's arrival and also serves as a lasting memory that you can both look back on and relive this amazing journey!

Depending on your preference, you can hire a professional photographer or simply have fun with just the two of you.

If you opt for the photographer, this gives you a chance to join in as well. Get creative and have fun!

Pro Tip:	Give mom plenty of notice for this shoot. Assume she will want to take the time to find the perfect outfit and have her hair done. This is her time to shine!

Push Present... Push it real good!

This term may be foreign to you, but it is most likely a very familiar one to your partner.

After enduring nine long months of hellish nausea, an out of control bladder, unbearable back pain, excruciating leg cramps, fireballs of heartburn (...and the list goes on ...) all leading up to the grueling marathon event of labor, some partners choose to gift moms with a present. Enter - "The Push Present".

Push presents usually come in the form of jewelry and relate back to your baby. For example, a necklace with a baby's foot, a bracelet that says your baby's name or a birthstone ring. But it can also be an experience such as a spa treatment for mom to enjoy when she is feeling up for it. Whichever you choose, make sure it is from the heart. At the end of the day, that is what matters to mom!

You can either give her the present before or after your baby is born. If you are superstitious, you may want to wait until after. Aim to make this an intimate moment for you and mom so you can express just how much you appreciate her.

28 Week Prenatal Appointment

The regular prenatal appointments will continue as per normal, the only difference being is that they are now biweekly. Expect to hear your baby's heartbeat and be sure to ask the doctor any questions or concerns you may have.

Week 28 Dad's Guide

Baby's Development

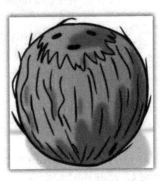

Size Estimate:

- Coconut
- Most babies begin shifting their bodies into a head-first downward position in preparation for birth in around 12 weeks. This is commonly considered the best position for a regular vaginal delivery and is otherwise known as 'cephalic presentation'.
- Baby may start becoming more active and mom may start to feel kicks and punches more regularly.

Pro Tip:	Some babies may not have turned face down by week 28, but don't worry it is still early days! The majority of babies will flip on their own over the next couple of months and if they don't, there are holistic methods to try such as yoga moves (more details at spinningbabies.com). If this is unsuccessful, a doctor may perform an external cephalic version (ECV) which is simply an attempt to turn your baby head down.

Mom's Changes

Physically:
New Symptoms:

- It might be time to pick up some bra pads as mom may be experiencing leaky breasts. This is normal and to be expected before your baby comes.

- As your baby continues growing, it begins to cramp some of mom's organs including her lungs, liver and intestines which may leave her with a shortness of breath.
- Baby is settling its way into the birthing position, which may involve them also touching mom's sciatic nerves. This can cause shooting pain down the back of her legs. Bed rest and warm compresses can help provide relief.

Recurring Symptoms:

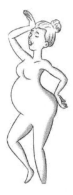

- Backaches, Braxton Hicks, stretch marks, heartburn, hemorrhoids, swollen hands and feet, trouble sleeping, constipation and leg cramps

Emotionally:

- The start of the third trimester can bring some pretty mixed emotions. The sense that meeting your baby is so near, is enough to fill her with both complete and utter joy and also some anxiety as well. The closer you get, the more these emotions may escalate.
- With the maternity photo shoot coming up, mom is most likely feeling herself! This is the perfect excuse to get all dressed up and let her hair down.

Dad's Feelings

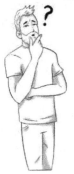

- You may be feeling pretty similar to mom this week. If you can remember when your baby was just 12 weeks and now has about 12 weeks left. Hold onto this feeling because the next few weeks are going to fly by!
- If the push present is purchased and ready to go, you are probably feeling pretty damn good. Pat yourself on the back. You did good, son, you did good!

Supporting Mom

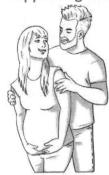

- Now that we're in the third trimester, be ready to book appointments bi-weekly, then weekly as the weeks progress!
- Double-check that the 30-week prenatal appointment is booked.

Important:	**Signs of preterm labor** – Although it is still very early on, if you see any of the following signs, be sure to call your doctor for further advice: - Mom's water breaks: a clear or colorless trickling discharge from mom's vagina that is not urine (normally has a sweet scent). - Strong contractions: strong pains in her stomach and back, repeating in a wave-like motion. - Mom feels baby 'suddenly' and/or abruptly dropping lower down into her pelvis.

Welcome to Week 29
Interviewing Pediatricians:
What's Up, Doc?

<u>TL, DR</u>: *A quick walkthrough guide on how to search for your baby's doctor.*

3 minute read

Fast facts covering:

- Finding a Pediatrician
- Important questions to ask

The Best Way to Find a Pediatrician

If you're looking for a good place to eat, you will usually ask around, get some feedback, check out some food porn pics, and then head to the eatery.

When you're looking for a pediatrician, you'll basically do the same (minus the porn pics of course).

Ask family and friends for honest feedback of doctors they've used for their children. From there, check out some online reviews. Then, call the office and schedule a tour.

Remember: even that very first call is the start of the interview. Note to yourself if you waited a while for someone to answer and was the receptionist hospitable?

Pro Tip:	Most clinics will offer "meet and greets" so you can get to know the doctors and support staff upfront. The

pediatrician you choose can also be your child's doctor until the age of 18. Make this a good choice!

What Should We Ask?

Just like the hospital tour - there are endless questions to ask but I have gone ahead and noted the most important:

- What was your initial gut feeling?
    - Not a question but crucial.
- Do you have privileges at the delivery hospital?
    - They will be the first doctors to come and meet your baby once born.
- Are same-day sick appointments a possibility? And is there a separate sick area in the waiting room?
    - You would want to avoid your newborn from being near other children with a cold while at the office.
- How are emergencies handled outside of working hours?
    - Is there a 24/7 doctor line to call?
- Are there any tests that a baby would need to be sent elsewhere for?

Week 29 Dad's Guide

Baby's Development

Size Estimate:

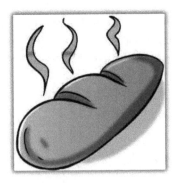

- Loaf of Bread (the closest to baked you'll be for a while)
- Baby's bones are hard at work this week getting stronger and stronger by the day.

- Baby's head is also increasing in size to accommodate their growing brain.

Pro Tip:	It's critical that mom continues eating calcium-rich foods because if your baby does not get enough calcium from mom's food consumption, they will take calcium directly from mom's bones, putting mom at risk of osteoporosis. Some examples are: dairy products, green leafy vegetables, pulses, tofu, orange juice and soybeans.

Mom's Changes

Physically:

Recurring Symptoms:

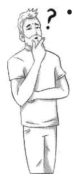

- Backaches, Braxton Hicks, RLS, stretch marks, heartburn, hemorrhoids, swollen hands and feet, itchy belly, trouble sleeping, constipation, leg cramps, shortness of breath, pregnancy brain, headaches, frequent urination and sciatic nerve pain.

Emotionally:

- Meeting the doctor who will care for your baby from birth is a huge deal! They will be the person you call in the middle of the night if your baby has a fever or their poop looks a little off. Deciding on who this person will be should help mom feel a great sense of relief!

Dad's Feelings

- You may be feeling like you are wearing many hats. From nutritionist (reminding mom what to eat and not to eat), masseuse (constant back and foot rubs), scholar (childbirth classes), secretary (making doctor appointments) and so on... This is totally normal and is something every dad should strive to do when possible. You are supporting mom and

161

helping her each day by doing these tasks and she will be forever grateful for your support.

Supporting Mom

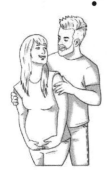

- Counting baby's kicks tends to start around this time. All it takes is reserving some time each day to count your baby's kicks whilst mom is seated or lying down. Ensure there are at least 10 movements over a one to two hour period. If baby isn't moving much, bring mom some icy cold water to drink, ask her to walk around a bit and then give her a massage before trying again. If there is still no movement and you are starting to feel concerned, you may want to consider calling your doctor for further advice.

Did You Know?	**Fetal Viability** - Although premature, according to studies, babies born at 29 weeks or later have a very strong survival rate of over 95%. Although you have now reached the somewhat safe zone, it is always best for babies to make it to 39-40 weeks full term, to ensure all organs are fully developed at birth.

Pro Tip:	**Pediatrician Visits** – Baby is normally scheduled in to see their new pediatrician within the first 7 days after birth. You should bring in baby's discharge papers and they generally get measured and weighed to create benchmarks for later examinations. Then, they usually go in for a monthly check up until month 3, at which point the visits will then move to every 3 months.

Welcome to Week 30
Childcare: *The Search Begins ...*

TL,DR: *Finding childcare while staying within your budget and comfort level.*

4 minute read

Fast facts covering:

- Childcare Options & Budgeting
- 30 Week Prenatal Appointment

If you haven't picked up on this trend yet, there are usually a lot of options for anything pregnancy or baby related. These span from where you have your baby, to what kind of crib to get, all the way to our new topic: Childcare.

Some parents require childcare if they will be returning to work after their allotted leave. It is never an easy decision to leave your baby, so the choice of who will be watching them is incredibly important.

You have three main options here:

Relatives
a) You know what they say, no one will love your child the way your family does. Or maybe my mom just says that... In any regard, this is usually the most comforting and affordable option. The downside here is, it may be hard to provide constructive feedback to them.
b) Cost - Typically free or very low cost.

Babysitter/Nanny
a) Babysitters can sometimes double as the nannies that not only watch your child but can also tidy up and cook. This is a

great option if you just want one main person with your child. But it can also be a negative if this one person is unavailable last minute.

b)   Cost - Babysitter's cost is usually higher than a relative depending on their duties (i.e. - are they also a nanny?)

Day care/School

a)   If you are interested in having your child socialize, this is a great option. The potential downside here is the number of germs they will be exposed to. Of course, this can also be a positive as it helps build their immune system.

b)   Cost – Day cares and schools are normally the highest cost.

Pro Tip:	**Save on Childcare Costs** – If work allows, both you and mom should enquire for the possibility of working from home, perhaps 1 or 2 days per week. This will certainly help save costs and/or reduce the reliance on relatives.

30 Week Prenatal Appointment

Expect to hear your baby's heartbeat and be sure to ask the doctor any questions or concerns you may have.

Week 30 Dad's Guide

Baby's Development

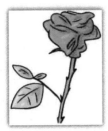

Size Estimate:

- Length of a short-stem rose (yes, go buy this for mom)
- Baby's hands are close to fully formed with fingernails under construction and baby's skin cells are starting to produce pigments forming your baby's skin color.

- Baby weighs around 3lbs and their brain is getting larger.
- If baby's head is not yet in a downward position, then it will happen very soon.

Mom's Changes

Physically:
Recurring Symptoms:

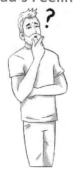

- Mom is likely to feel baby's movement every day now and they are most commonly felt after a meal or when resting in a seated or lying down position.
- Backaches, Braxton Hicks, fatigue, mood changes, breast sensitivity, bloating, stretch marks, heartburn, hemorrhoids, swollen hands and feet, trouble sleeping, constipation, leg cramps, shortness of breath, frequent urination and sciatic nerve pain.

Emotionally:

- Mom may be dealing with some insensitive comments that can be making her feel insecure. Such as "WOW, are you carrying twins" or "You're still pregnant?!". The best thing for mom to do is to let these roll down her sore sweaty back and just smile.

Dad's Feelings

- You still haven't even met your child, but you have already started to look for someone to watch them. Putting your trust in someone can be worrisome. It is totally normal to feel apprehensive about this. Listen to your heart and rely on your gut. It will get easier as the days progress.

Supporting Mom

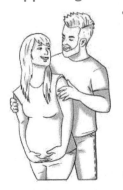

- Keep mom feeling confident! It can be difficult for her to see her body changing while dealing with so many pregnancy symptoms. If she is receiving similar insensitive comments as mentioned above, she will really need you to balance those out with some positivity. Remind her how beautiful she is every day and tell her that her skin is glowing!
- Double-check that the 32-week prenatal appointment is booked.

Did You Know?	Some hospitals do not allow you to leave with your newborn baby unless you have a car seat already installed. Yep, you heard right! So if you haven't already, get to researching car seats asap as baby is just around the corner!

Celebrate Pregnancy:	An idea to commemorate mom's pregnancy and celebrate her growing belly in style is to suggest booking in a "Henna Belly Art" session. If mom is interested in this, be sure to book an artist who uses 100% natural henna dye which is derived from henna trees. Another alternative to henna is a "Pregnancy Belly Cast". These can be a fun, quick and an affordable DIY project for you both to bond. The plaster sets around mom's belly in as little as 15 minutes to form a belly cast and it captures mom's beautiful bump which can then be displayed as a commemorative piece of home décor!

Welcome to Week 31
Parental Leave: *Sayonara Suckers!*

TL,DR: *Discuss parental leave with your employer and ask key questions on company policies.*

Important Note:	Your manager should be made aware of your upcoming plan to leave prior to 31 weeks. This should be shared usually around the same time you announce it to your friends and family, which we covered in week 12. So around 31 weeks, is typically when you confirm your parental leave and meet with Human Resources (HR).

4 minute read

Fast facts covering:

- Parental Leave & Company Policies
- Discussion points you need to have

There is no hard or fast rule on the amount of time you are able to take off from work and whether it will be fully paid or not. You may be offered parental leave depending on factors such as where you live and your company's specific policies. Therefore, it is usually best to meet with your Human Resource Team and manager to review your options.

For instance - in the state of New York, FMLA (family medical leave act) allows you to take leave as either the primary caregiver or secondary caregiver. The mother is typically primary, and the father is secondary, and leave usually ranges from 8 to 16 weeks. On the other hand, if your company is small (less than 50 employees), there *may not* be an option for leave or it may be very minimal. Again, everyone's situation is different, so it is best to consult with your employer directly.

Important Questions

Sometimes it is best to let your HR team explain the benefits first, then dive in with your questions after. They may offer more than you thought. Some items to cover are:

- Do I need to file for leave or does the company do that for me?
- What if I need more time, what are my options for extending leave?
- How would I go about adding my child to my company health insurance and benefits so he or she is covered right after birth?
- While on leave, do I have access to log in and check work?
- When I do return, is there a flexible transition schedule or straight back to regular hours?

Week 31 Dad's Guide

Baby's Development

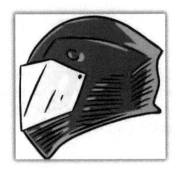

Size Estimate:

- Motorcycle Helmet (sell the bike before your kid comes or up that life insurance!)
- Baby is likely to double in weight over the next 9 weeks!
- Crazy to imagine but all of your baby's five senses are now activated as they can now hear, taste, touch, smell, and see!

Mom's Changes

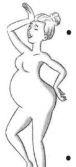

Physically:
Recurring Symptoms:

- Backaches, Braxton Hicks, pregnancy brain, stretch marks, backaches, heartburn, leaky breasts, hemorrhoids, swollen hands and feet, trouble sleeping, constipation, leg cramps, shortness of breath, frequent urination, sciatic nerve pain, and general discomfort

Emotionally:

- Mom has most likely told her job as well about parental leave. She may be swamped with meetings to help make her transition out of work easier. Hopefully, mom is feeling some relief from this!

Dad's Feelings

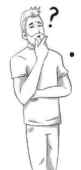

- Nothing throws you more into a reality check like setting a pending deadline for work to end and parental leave to begin. This makes it even more real!

Supporting Mom

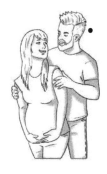

- Start prepping your baby's nursery. A lot of the big-ticket items may not arrive until your baby shower (if you haven't had it yet), but you can get started on other things such as: painting or washable wallpapering, adding curtains or blinds (blackout curtains to mimic nighttime for the win!), hanging decor, etc.

169

Pro Tip: If mom is experiencing a shortness of breath, it may continue until baby drops lower down into mom's pelvis. When your baby drops this is also known as 'dropping' or 'lightening'. This can happen anywhere from 2-6 weeks before delivery and is a sign that mom's body is preparing for labor! Once this happens mom should find it easier to breath, however since your baby is now lower down, the pressure on mom's bladder will trigger more bathroom stops! (once baby's head is down, this feeling can be described as though they are hauling around a bowling ball between mom's thighs!)

Heads Up: A very nice gesture that mom will really appreciate is if you book in a manicure and pedicure session for her! This is because around this time many pregnant women experience dry and brittle nails, so come in and save the day with this perfect surprise!

Month 7 Checklist & Reminders
(Because who has time to make their own list?)

☐   Purchase a push present

☐   Schedule the maternity photoshoot

☐   Start counting kicks

☐   Find a Pediatrician

☐   Decide on childcare

☐   Set up Parental Leave

☐   Schedule 32 & 34-week prenatal appointments

MONTH 8 - Weeks 32 through 35
Learn about:

- **Packing Hospital Bag:** *what you'll need to get through the stay*

- **Setting up Nursery:** *let's get creative, dad!*

- **Properly Installing Car Seat:** *and get it approved, too*

- **Feeding Baby:** *breastfeeding, bottle feeding, or formula*

- **Signs of Labor:** *what to look for when labor approaches*

Let's Paint the Picture:
Baby's Nursery

Wife's instructions - *Pick up a can of purple paint.*

Sounds easy enough. Though as I stand in the paint aisle, I realize purple is not simply purple. It's periwinkle, grape soda, mauve, Barney, voodoo daiquiri, lavender, lilac and sangria... I mistakenly thought there would be a stand-alone can labeled "Purple" waiting on a shelf of its own.

I debate calling my wife and decide against it. She asked me to do one favor today, and god willing, I will get it done. Plus, she has the big job. You know the one where she pushes a pumpkin sized baby out of an incredibly small hole? But hey, I'm contributing. I'm about to paint a nursery. Well, I guess saying it aloud pales in comparison.

Time to make a game time decision. I opt for an ever-so sophisticated round of Eeny, Meeny, Miny, Moe - the decision is made. Lilac it is.

I arrive home and head up the stairs and to the left towards the nursery. As I get closer, I hear what seems to be The Electric Slide blaring from inside. Sure enough, it is. And there she is - my darling wife, wearing a pair of Dungarees overalls.

She means business.

My wife's belly, once reserved solely as our daughter's humble abode, doubles as a paintbrush holder for the day. We spend hours painting the nursery and laugh about the color. The music changes from the late 80's wedding jams, to current R&B hits.

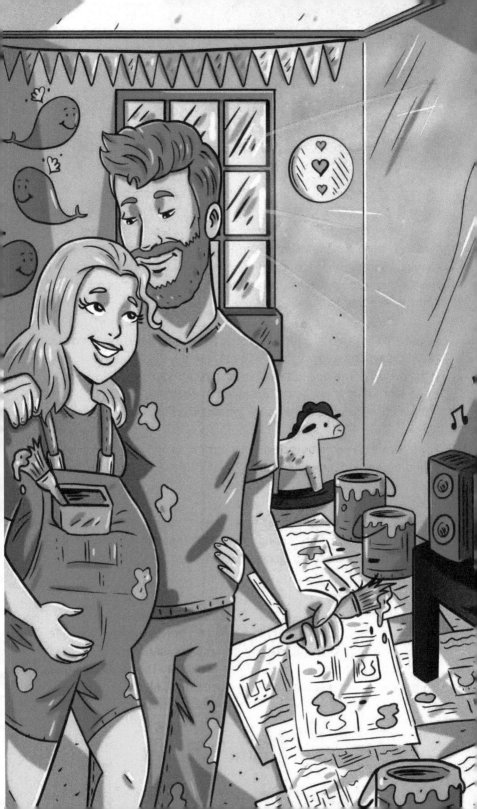

Now it's a party.

As the sun shines in on our lilac shaded room, I think to myself this is arguably the most perfect day. My wife leans back into my arms and at that moment I realize how lucky this baby is to have my wife as her mother and how lucky we are to have each other.

Welcome to Week 32
Hospital Preparation:
Bags Packed & Ready To Go!

__*TL, DR*__: *Get your hospital bag ready with essentials such as clothes, toiletries and snacks.*

3 minute read

Fast facts covering:

- Packing the Hospital Bag
- 34 Week Prenatal Appointment

Peek over at your partner's pregnancy reading material and you'll be sure to find lists about what mom needs to pack for the hospital stay. But, what you most likely won't find are lists dedicated to just dad. Instead of guessing what to pack or asking your partner, take the lead here!

What goes in the bag?

Clothes:

- Two to three comfortable outfits for the day such as sweatpants or jeans with a t-shirt
- Hoodie or sweater since the hospital's temperature fluctuates
- Flip flops to use in the shower

Toiletries:

- Shampoo, conditioner and body wash
- Contacts and/or glasses
- Toothbrush and toothpaste

Food:

- Non-refrigerated snacks such as granola, breakfast bars and crackers
- Water or sports drinks

Misc:

- Push present if you plan to give it after labor
- Phone charger

Pro Tip:	Leave the bags in your car or right by your door. Easy to spot and grab when it's time!

32 Week Prenatal Appointment

Expect to hear your baby's heartbeat and be sure to ask the doctor any questions or concerns you may have.

Week 32 Dad's Guide

Baby's Development

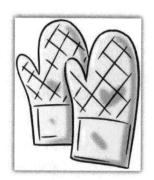

Size Estimate:
- **Pair of Oven Mitts** (have them ready as your bun is nearly done!)
- Your baby can focus on objects that are close-range and this ability to focus will stay that way until birth.
- All of baby's vital organs are now completely formed apart from the lungs and if they were born this week, chances of survival are very high.

Mom's Changes

Physically:

New Symptoms:

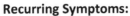

- Mom may be able to breathe a bit easier now that baby is dropping lower into her pelvis and releasing the pressure off her diaphragm.

Recurring Symptoms:

- Backaches, Braxton Hicks (increased intensity & frequency), stretch marks, heartburn, hemorrhoids, swollen hands and feet, trouble sleeping, constipation, dizziness, leaky breasts, itchy belly/skin, and leg cramps

Emotionally:

- 32 Weeks can be an odd time for mom. It is before 36 weeks which typically signifies that your baby can come at any point, but it's within the third trimester. This time of limbo can cause mom to feel anxious about what is to come, but also impatient waiting for it.

Heads Up:	If mom hasn't experienced much back pain throughout pregnancy and is suddenly feeling it now, this could be a sign of preterm labor, so it's best to contact your doctor for further advice if this happens.

Symptom Relievers:	**Back Aches** – Perform Pelvic Tilt exercises. Mom stands with her back to the wall and presses the arch of her lower back into the wall. Can also be done on the floor. Repeat for 3-5 minutes.

Itchy Skin / Belly - Massage Anti-itch lotions & Cocoa Butter or Vitamin E Moisturizers onto the affected |

areas whilst mom's skin is moist (e.g. after bathing). This helps trap the moisture into her skin.

Supporting Mom

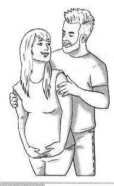

- You've packed your bag for the hospital, now what if you also packed mom's bag as well. Take the initiative here. Review what's in the bag with your partner before putting it in the car... You wouldn't want to forget an essential item you didn't realize was important.
- Double-check that the 34-week prenatal appointment is booked.

Pro Tips:

1. Inform your health insurance company that your partner is pregnant and to add baby to your policy. You may also need to provide them with the birth certificate and normally have 30 days after birth to get this done.

2. Finalise your birth plan so you can both share it with your doctor. When labor does strike, you need to be confident and strong in the delivery room and make sure that (where possible), mom's wishes on the birth plan don't deviate too much and are followed as closely as can be.

Important:

Look out for ... Mucus Plug and Water Discharge – The mucus plug looks like a thick, slimy, white-ish or yellow-ish (and sometimes slightly bloody), gooey discharge. You need to ensure mom is monitoring for this and/or a constant leaking watery discharge (not urine), which could indicate her waters are breaking. If either occurs, call your doctor immediately for further advice.

Welcome to Week 33
Finalize To-Do List & Baby Shower
Over – *Check!*

_TL,DR_: *Check for baby registry items you still need, set up the nursery and install the car seat!*

5 minute read

Fast facts covering:

- Double-check registry items
- Nursery set up
- Car seat installation & Hospital rules

The baby shower may be behind you, but the to-do list is glaring at you from across the room. Let's get started on it, shall we?

First on the list, checking the baby registry items you received with the items you requested. Ask yourself, was this what we really wanted? If the answer is no, then return it. Most stores will have a pretty flexible return policy. If you asked for some items but didn't receive them, now would be a good time to pick those up.

Project nursery underway

Ahh, maybe you imagined the nursery being space-themed or jungle fever! Maybe you never really gave it much thought before. Wherever you are, it's time to give it some thought! Get creative! Have fun with different colors and themes. If this is your first child, enjoy the task of creating their first room.

You can take a bit more time thinking of those finishing touches, but this week, focus on building the crib, putting together the dresser, and organizing baby's clothes. Decide how you plan to cancel out noise (such as a sound machine) and get the changing table prepped with diapers and plenty of wipes! Aim to have the nursery complete by 36 weeks in case of an early arrival!

Strap that baby in!

You will need a baby's car seat installed prior to leaving the hospital, so let's get going on this safety-first item. It may seem like you're reading a totally foreign language when trying to decipher how one even installs a car seat. Why are there so many straps and do we really need five pages of instructions?

Give it your best shot and keep in mind that in most areas your local fire station will check that the car seat was installed properly for you! This is usually a free, quick and painless process that involves pulling up to a fire station and having them check all the safety points on it. Call around to check what your local fire stations offer.

Did You Know?	Depending on where you live and your hospital's policies, you may not be able to leave the hospital without a car seat installed. In fact, most hospitals require you to bring the car seat in before leaving so they can see you strap your baby in safely!

For those who don't own a car - you may wish to consider asking family/friends or hiring a taxi/rideshare, but make sure the cars are equipped with a baby car seat. Other options are public transport or simply walking (if nearby!).

Remember, be sure to check as each hospital's policy is different.

Week 33 Dad's Guide

Baby's Development

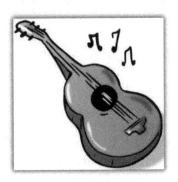

Size Estimate:

- A Small Ukulele (it's popular in some regions!)
- A new milestone reached as baby now has their own immune system!

Fun Fact:	Baby's skull bones are still quite malleable and not fully hardened. This allows baby to squeeze their head through mom's birth canal which is the reason why some newborns have "coneheads" for the first few days!

Mom's Changes

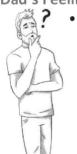

Physically:
Recurring Symptoms:

- Backaches, Braxton Hicks, stretch marks, heartburn, hemorrhoids, swollen hands and feet, trouble sleeping, constipation and leg cramps.

Emotionally:

- If your baby shower has passed, mom is probably feeling incredibly loved. There's nothing like a room full of loved ones to shower mom with compliments, presents, and great food!

Dad's Feelings

- Once items start coming off of the good old "honey-do list", the anxiety starts to disappear a bit for dad. When that last screw is nailed into the crib, and that last strap is fastened into the car seat, you should be feeling one step closer to getting ready to welcome that baby!

Supporting Mom

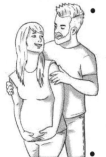

- Does anyone really enjoy writing thank you notes? I'm going to go with an astounding no! This week, you may want to tackle those baby shower thank-you's. If you don't have the best handwriting, accompany your partner while she writes them. A little humor and good attitude will help pass the time as she writes "we appreciate the thoughtful gift!" 30 times.
- Book the 34-week prenatal appointment.

Pro Tip:	Be proactive and finish assembling that baby gear (i.e. crib, stroller etc.) in advance and even before mom asks! If you find the instructions difficult to follow, jump on YouTube and type the model number in or speak to the retailer for advice.

Reminders:	1. Wash all of baby's clothes well in advance of their arrival, to ensure they are nice and clean and free from any residual chemicals and potential skin irritants from the factory. Look for washing detergents specifically for sensitive skin that are suitable for babies. 2. Double check that the hospital (or birth centre) has successfully confirmed your registration.

Welcome to Week 34
Feeding Baby: *Got Milk?*

TL, DR: *Deciding how you want to feed your baby (breast, bottle or formula)*

5 minute read

Fast facts covering:

- Methods for Feeding Baby
- 34 Week Prenatal Appointment

When it comes to feeding your baby there are a few methods to choose from, and your choice really depends on what you and your partner are comfortable with. From zero to six months, it is normally recommended that babies drink milk as their main food source.

Below are the options for milk consumption:

- Breastfeeding (aka 'Nursing')
- Breast Pumping and then Bottle Feeding
- Formula Bottle Feeding

The American Academy of Pediatrics suggests breast milk as the best source, but this is a huge commitment for mom and may not always be a feasible option.

There are many reasons why some moms choose not to nurse such as mom having a low milk supply, having to return to work or simply because formula may be their preference.

After six months of age you can slowly introduce foods starting with purees and then gradually work your way through to solids.

34 Week Prenatal Appointment

Expect to hear your baby's heartbeat and be sure to ask the doctor any questions or concerns you may have.

Week 34 Dad's Guide

Baby's Development

Size Estimate:

- Blender (for those nights you're craving a juice)
- Watch closely as you may be able to see your baby's tiny hands and feet kicking through mom's stomach!

- Around this week is when baby's finger and toenails have fully grown onto their hands and feet. Baby may require a clip not too long after their debut, so be sure to add baby nail clippers to your shopping list. Hot tip - One of the best times to cut their nails is whilst they are asleep, otherwise they can tend to constantly flail their arms and legs about making it a very difficult task!

Mom's Changes

Physically:
Recurring Symptoms:

- Backaches, Braxton Hicks, stretch marks, heartburn, hemorrhoids, swollen hands and feet, trouble sleeping, constipation, and leg cramps.

Emotionally:

- Around week 34, most moms will agree that they've had enough. From the recurring symptoms that add to their discomforts, to their growing belly - they may just want delivery day to come already!

Supporting Mom

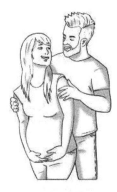

- Baby sneak peak - Have you ever seen a 3D or 4D baby scan? It is basically a way more detailed ultrasound showing what your baby looks like including their facial features and you may even catch them blinking and/or smiling at you! Depending on the service provider, you can normally take away photos (and videos) of the session.
To top that, these 3D scans can then be converted into a 3D life-like model of your unborn baby, which you can keep as a precious memento! How cool is that?!
- After seeking your doctor's approval, why not book in a session for you and mom. These are normally done at specialized ultrasound facilities and a quick internet search in your local area should point you in the right direction.

Pro Tips:	**Test Run:** Perform a test run to the hospital including planning of alternate routes such as back streets. The last thing you want is getting stuck in peak hour traffic or unplanned road work delays when it's go-time! **Shopping Run:** It's a good idea to have your pantry stocked up with staples and essentials in preparation for baby's arrival. Schedule in a big grocery shop and remember to also buy any final baby supplies such as wipes, diapers, clothing, etc.

Welcome to Week 35
Signs Of Labor:
Keep Doc On Standby!

TL, DR: *What to look out for when labor is near: baby drops, contractions increase, water breaks and more...*

4 minute read

Fast facts covering:

- Signs of Labor Approaching

They say, when a woman is in labor, they know it. But what about before real labor sets in. What signs should you look for? Well - a few actually!

- **Increased vaginal discharge or the "bloody show"**
    - Yup, the bloody show. It's exactly what it sounds like - discharge with blood. Not to be mistaken for a really great horror movie.
- **Contractions begin to feel more intense**
    - Mom will be able to tell the true difference between Braxton Hicks and regular contractions here.
- **Water breaks**
    - When mom's water breaks, labor is pretty imminent. Though, the majority of the time the water is broken by a doctor at the hospital to speed up labor.
- **Diarrhea can increase leading up to labor**
    - This allows mom's body to clear the way for baby!
- **Baby drops into the birth canal**
    - This is a visual change that you will probably notice with mom's belly being lower, and a physical change for her as she will be able to breathe a bit better.

Week 35 Dad's Guide

Baby's Development

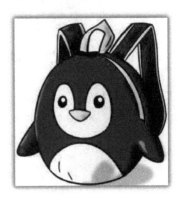

Size Estimate:

- Kid's Backpack (preparing you for the future)

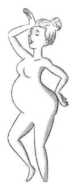

- Most babies are now in the head down position ready for a regular vaginal delivery.
- The amniotic fluid surrounding baby will start to diminish over the coming weeks.
- Baby is still gaining weight and building up their own body fat which keeps their body warm and regulates their temperature.

Mom's Changes

Physically:
Recurring Symptoms:

- Backaches, Braxton Hicks, stretch marks, heartburn, hemorrhoids, swollen hands and feet, trouble sleeping, constipation, and leg cramps.

Emotionally:

- Mom may be feeling really excited at this time as she sees the finish line in sight. She can really go into labor at any point from week 36 onwards. So, this last week is right before things really pick up!

Dad's Feelings

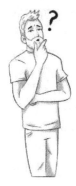

- You may be feeling overwhelmed with all the last-minute checks and preparation required into getting ready for baby's debut. Don't stress too much. Remember to ensure you have the essentials done including: a place for baby to safely sleep, car seat installed and inspected by professionals and baby basics like clothing, diapers and wipes. Take peace in knowing you've got all the absolute essentials ticked off!

Did You Know?	An estimated 85-90% of baby car seats are not installed correctly! An alarming statistic considering this is what keeps your baby safe. After installation, be sure to have your car seat inspected by a qualified technician at your baby store or fire station, this is normally a free service.

Supporting Mom

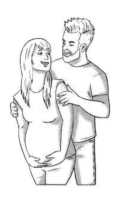

- It's not too early to prepare for labor signs. As a heads up, you usually want to head to the hospital when mom's contractions follow the 311 rule, meaning they occur every three minutes, last one minute, and continue for one hour long. Take the lead and download a contraction timing mobile app, allowing you to count from the start of one contraction to the start of the next. Alternatively, you can also jot down the frequency of contractions on paper by referring to a clock or stopwatch. So when labor does strike, you'll be prepared and know exactly what to do!
- Double-check that the 36-week prenatal appointment is booked.

Pro Tips:

1. Baby has most likely moved into a head down position by this stage which is most suited for delivery. However, a small percentage (around 2-4%) of baby's assume a 'breech' position, which means their legs are pointing downward. This can cause complications for birth, but don't worry too much, as most baby's normally still flip into a head down position in the last few weeks in time for delivery. If baby is still not head down, one way to encourage baby to shift is for mom to go on regular walks. This can help work baby's head downwards into mom's pelvis due to the forces of gravity and the motion of her hips swaying side to side.

2. Keep Mom Hydrated! Even though mom is continually running to the bathroom every 5 minutes, ensure she stays well hydrated, as dehydration can actually bring on preterm labor, putting your baby's health at risk.

Discussion Point:

Consider Cord Blood Banking – this is the blood that's left over in the placenta and umbilical cord after birth. This blood contains stem cells that can help treat certain diseases such as some cancers. It can be kept by you and used at a later stage if someone in your family is diagnosed with a treatable disease or alternatively, can be donated to a public cord blood bank. This is generally a painless and easy procedure taking no more than 10 minutes.

Twin Pregnancies:

Although full term for twins is normally 37-38 weeks, a large portion of twin pregnancies are born around 36 weeks (or sometimes earlier).

Month 8 Checklist & Reminders
(Because who has time to make their own list?)

☐   Pack the hospital bag

☐   Get creative with baby's nursery

☐   Send baby shower thank you notes

☐   Install the car seat & get it approved!

☐   Double-check that weeks 36 through 40 prenatal appointments are booked.

MONTH 9 - Weeks 36 through 42
Learn about:

⁺ **Pain Relief Options**: *natural and medicated labor assistance*

⁺ **Pregnancy Terms**: *from pre-term to post-term*

⁺ **Nesting**: *time to childproof and clean*

⁺ **Inductions & C-Sections**: *learning about alternative options*

⁺ **Going Past Due Date**: *and fielding family members' and friends' labor inquires*

Month 9 Checklist & Reminders
(Brought forward in case your baby arrives early!)

☐   Familiarize yourself with pain relief options

☐   Watch in amazement as your partner frantically cleans the house and prepares for baby

    ☐   Then help her and join along in the joy of nesting

☐   Childproof your home

☐   Research induction stories to gain varying perspectives on the experience

☐   Consider alternative delivery options such as a c-section, inductions, forceps and a vacuum procedure

☐   Enjoy some one on one time with your partner

☐   Practice patience as you wait for your baby to arrive

☐   Make a 41-week appointment if you go past the due date

Let's Paint the Picture:
Inducing Labor

Maybe we should try that new Indian spot tonight and have sex."

My wife sheepishly asks me this on the car ride home. On any other occasion, both of those options would have been wonderful! But I'll admit, I'm hesitant to... Lay down the pipe... with my wife being so pregnant. Then there's the Indian food which combined with her heartburn, might not be a good idea.

She tells me that spicy foods and semen will help induce labor. I tell her, what wifey wants, wifey gets.

We get home and are off to the races.

Laying down next to each other feels like old times. As she moves the sheet back, I see her belly and I'm reminded that this will be different than the old times.

We spend a good five to ten minutes trying to maneuver the best position without her belly blocking the goalie. The end result is her on top and me as giddy as I'd never been before to have sex with my wife.

The deed is done and by noon the next day, my wife starts having light contractions. She smiles at me from across the room and thanks me for taking one for the team.

Little does she know, I'm the best team player and am happy to be tagged in anytime, anywhere.

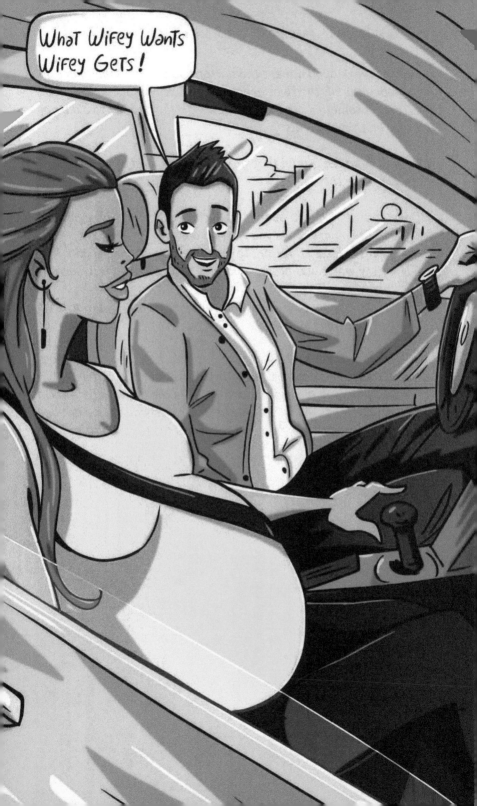

At our 41-week appointment the doctor told us that if we didn't go into labor naturally then we needed to schedule an induction for week 42. There is something about the word induction that evokes a bit of fear for first-time parents.

Maybe it's the realization that there is an actual deadline and your baby will come then.

Or the fact that if you search "induction stories" they're usually negative. The main themes you will find are:

- *"Labor lasted three entire days after the Pitocin injection"*
- *"My water was broken and then labor came to a screeching halt"*
- *"Extremely painful contractions right from the get-go with zero rest in between.*

You see what I mean - nothing positive. We had to do a bit more digging to find the really awesome stories about it. The ones from moms who praised the process and thanked the heavens for Pitocin and Foley Bulbs. As the induction was already scheduled, we decided then and there that we were only going to focus on those positive stories...

Welcome to Week 36
Pain Relief Options:
Hook Me Up, Doctor!

TL, DR: *There are many pain relief options for moms that are both natural and medicated. These range from breathing techniques, to an epidural.*

4 minute read

Fast facts covering:

- Pain Relief Options During Labor
- 36 Week Prenatal Appointment
  - Group B Strep Test
  - Checking Dilation & Effacement

Have you ever been kicked in the testicles before and been told by a woman that compared to childbirth, that it's a walk in the park? I have... twice. And both times I thought, well, sure if the park is a torture chamber and the walk is over a field of knives.

That all changed when my wife was in labor. I'll take that walk in the park any day.

So, what can a mom do to help her through labor? She has two main routes: natural and medicated.

Natural:

- Breath it out. Try hypnobirthing which is a method for breathing and relaxing your body during painful contractions.
- Put on some music, a tv show or a movie on a portable device. This can help to distract and relax mom during labor.

- Massage mom to distract her from the pain and apply a warm compress to release natural painkilling endorphins.

- Light some incense or essential oils which are used as natural relaxants.

Medicated:

- Epidural. By far the most popular method of pain relief. This is administered through a needle in mom's back effectively numbing the lower half of her body.
- Laughing gas is a mask that mom puts on her mouth and can inhale when she needs relief from pain and/or anxiety.

36 Week Prenatal Appointment & Beyond

During this week's appointment, mom will have a Group B Strep Test done to check for bacteria that can cause infection in the placenta and amniotic fluid. If mom tests positive, she will need antibiotics given every 4 hours during labor to protect your baby.

Another new task that will be performed from week 36 up until delivery is checking for dilation and effacement. Dilating (or opening up) is from 1 - 10cm and effacement (or thinning out) is measured from 0-100%. Both are measurements used to determine if there is a large enough passage for baby to pass through. This check involves the doctor inserting his fingers into mom's vagina to see how she is progressing. Some women are against this procedure and refuse to have them, as they really can't guarantee when your baby will come. A woman can be 4cm dilated (opened) and 80% effaced (thinned out) for weeks, whereas another woman could be 1cm dilated and 50% effaced and go into labor that same day. Another reason for refusal is that the procedure may cause an infection if bacteria enters the vagina.

After week 36, appointments will begin to occur weekly in order to closely watch your baby's health.

Week 36 Dad's Guide

Baby's Development

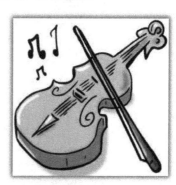

Size Estimate:

- A Violin (serenade your partner)
- Although baby will still continue gaining weight, their rapid rate of growth will begin to

slow down, allowing baby to fit through the birth canal for delivery. This will also allow mom to build up and reserve energy stores for the big day!
- Baby's immune system has been fully developed and is able to fight off outside world viruses, bacteria and infections. However, their digestive system is not yet ready to fully function and may take up to 1-2 years outside of the womb to be in full operation. The reason for the lag is that baby has relied heavily on mom's placenta and umbilical cord to supply nutrients, and therefore their digestive system has not yet been in operation.

Mom's Changes

Physically:

- By now, mom may have substituted walking with something that resembles more of a "penguin waddle".
- Mom's ligaments, joints and connective tissues are loosening, allowing baby to more easily squeeze through during delivery.

Recurring Symptoms:

- Backaches, Braxton Hicks, stretch marks, heartburn, hemorrhoids, swollen hands and feet, trouble sleeping, constipation, and leg cramps.

Emotionally:

- Mom will have taken her Step B test around week 36 and she will need to wait a few days to find out the results. Even if she tests positive, it won't change the pregnancy. Keep mom calm!

Dad's Feelings

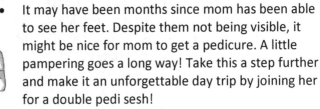

- The first thing you're likely to hear at the doctor's visit is that your baby can come at any point from here. Try not to worry or panic! You've checked off some pretty big items if your baby did come now. You are prepared. If you are still feeling anxious about the impending labor, it is totally normal. Just take a deep breath and know you've got this, Dad!

Supporting Mom

- It may have been months since mom has been able to see her feet. Despite them not being visible, it might be nice for mom to get a pedicure. A little pampering goes a long way! Take this a step further and make it an unforgettable day trip by joining her for a double pedi sesh!
- Double-check that the 37-week prenatal appointment is booked.

Reminder:	As mentioned in week 32, remind mom to keep an eye out for signs of her mucus plug being released. If it makes an appearance, consult your doctor immediately for further advice.

Twin Pregnancies:	Although most twins are usually born by around week 36-37, they are normally in good health. Twin pregnancies consider 38 weeks as full term as opposed to 40 weeks for singleton babies.

Welcome to Week 37
'Term' Stages Of Pregnancy:
How Long Is Your Bun In The Oven?

TL, DR: *Becoming familiar with pregnancy terms related to pre-term labor all the way to the post-term labor.*

Important Note:	Check out Chapter 10 for the '3 Stages of Labor and Delivery' ahead of time, so you know what to expect when mom goes into labor - *as it may be before her due date!*

4 minute read

Fast facts covering:

- Different 'Term' Levels
- 37 Week Prenatal Appointment

Going into labor either *before* or *after* your due date is much more common than going into labor *on* your actual due date. If you fall into that bucket, it will be helpful to know which term level your baby falls into. Babies born on the following weeks are categorized as follows:

- Before 37 weeks, 0 days   = **Pre**-term (or Premature)
  Between:
  - 37 weeks, 0 days and 38 weeks, 6 days
                        = **Early**-term
  - 39 weeks, 0 days and 40 weeks, 6 days
                        = **Full**-term
  - 41 weeks, 0 days and 41 weeks, 6 days
                        = **Late**-term

- After 42 weeks, 0 days   =   **Post**-term

If your baby is born early-term, they may have issues with breathing and feeding at the start. Despite this, the majority end up living full and healthy lives. They may just need to spend some time in NICU (neonatal intensive care unit). NICU is the area in hospitals that specializes in caring for newborns that may require some extra attention.

37 Week Prenatal Appointment

Expect to hear your baby's heartbeat and be sure to ask the doctor any questions or concerns you may have.

Week 37 Dad's Guide

Baby's Development

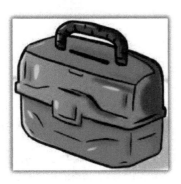

Size Estimate:

- Fishing Tackle Box (a great father-child pastime)
- Baby may be sucking on their fingers in preparation for feeding outside of the womb!
- Baby's hair is mostly grown by this stage and at birth may actually be a different color to you and your partners. But sometimes this color is only temporary and their hair may fall out and regrow their true color.

Mom's Changes

Physically:

New Symptoms:

- Pelvic Pain – Mom may experience new pelvic pains due to baby's head nestling deeper into her pelvic area in preparation for birth.

Pro Tip: To help mom relieve pelvic pains, there are a few options: Prepare a warm bath for her, give her pain points a massage (or book in a prenatal massage), instruct her to perform some pelvic exercises such as Kegels or try a pregnancy belly band for some added support.

New Symptoms:

- Mom may notice some "spotting" or a couple of drops of blood around this time which is usually quite normal. However, if it is more than a few spots, then consult your doctor immediately.

Recurring Symptoms:

- Backaches, Braxton Hicks (increased intensity and frequency), stretch marks, heartburn, hemorrhoids, swollen hands and feet, trouble sleeping, constipation, dizziness, leaky breasts, itchy belly/skin, and leg cramps.

Emotionally:

- Most moms will want their labor to begin prior to their due date. They're over being so pregnant and want to meet their baby. However once learning the term levels and what they each mean for baby's development, moms may think otherwise and be okay with the baby hanging out a little longer. This can be an emotional roller coaster for a mom who is torn between the two. Generally speaking, the longer your baby stays inside the womb, the more developed the will be.

Supporting Mom

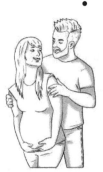

- How many poopy diapers have you and mom changed in your day? If the answer is less than 5, then you might want to spend some time together practicing those diaper changes. This can be a really fun activity to do with mom to help pass the time when waiting for your baby. To put a spin on this, put a diaper on a doll but have it move around, a lot! Time each other, make it a competition! Friendly, of course. The winner gets a back rub. (PS - mom gets the back rub regardless!)
- Double-check that the 38-week prenatal appointment is booked.

Reminder:	**Be Prepared** – Did you know that less than 5% of babies are born on their due dates? Be prepared for baby to come any time now and ensure you have ticked off all the essentials on your to-do list!

Pro Tips:	**1. Get An Exercise Ball** – A great way for mom to exercise this late into her pregnancy is an exercise (or birthing) ball. These can help mom perform safe stretches, strengthen her core muscles and is also another alternative for natural pain relief during labor.
	2. Practice Using Baby Devices – Familiarize yourself with essential baby gear such as the car seat (which should be installed and inspected by now). It's probably one of the first devices you will use and as mentioned, you'll most likely need one fitted before you're allowed to take baby home! Ensure you're familiar with all the different adjustment settings and safety features.

Welcome to Week 38
Nesting & Childproofing:
A Baby-Friendly Home

TL, DR: *The nesting instinct kicks in, which leads to lots of cleaning and baby preparation such as childproofing.*

Important Note:	Check out Chapter 10 for the '3 Stages of Labor and Delivery' ahead of time, so you know what to expect when mom goes into labor - *as it may be before her due date!*

4 minute read

Fast facts covering:

- Nesting Instinct
- Childproofing Your Home
- 38 Week Prenatal Appointment

Nesting is simply an instinct to prepare for your baby's arrival. You may find your partner rummaging around the house, and you may find yourself doing the same! This includes cleaning, laundry, organizing the home and double-checking baby items.

Go with it! Who doesn't love a clean house and some baby prep!

While at it, take some time to check the below items and also start childproofing unsafe areas where necessary:

- Carbon Monoxide
  - Install detectors or check battery levels
- First Aid

- o   Keep an emergency kit in the house and in the car
- Fire Control
  - o   Ensure fire extinguishers are handy
  - o   Check batteries in smoke detectors
- Furniture
  - o   Round off any sharp edges or corners with bumpers

38 Week Prenatal Appointment

Expect to hear your baby's heartbeat and be checked for dilation and effacement if mom opted for this. Be sure to ask the doctor any questions or concerns you may have.

Week 38 Dad's Guide

Baby's Development

Size Estimate:

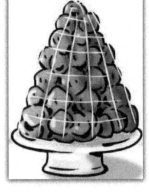

- Croquembouche (go ahead, look up the recipe)

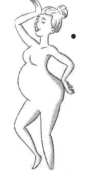

- Apart from baby continuing to put on weight in the form of body fat, all other developmental milestones have been reached and it is simply a wait for mother nature to run its course!

Mom's Changes

Physically:

Recurring Symptoms:

- Backaches, Braxton Hicks (increased intensity and frequency), stretch marks, heartburn, hemorrhoids, swollen hands and feet, trouble sleeping, constipation, dizziness, leaky breasts, itchy belly/skin, and leg cramps.

Emotionally:

- Mom has most likely had Braxton Hicks for a while now. But as the due date approaches, every little twinge can feel like the real thing. Due to this, mom may be feeling more mentally exhausted than usual and waking up throughout the night overthinking what each slight pain or movement might signify.

Dad's Feelings

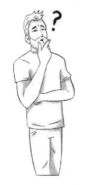

- With two weeks left until the due date, you may be reflecting on the type of dad you want to be. It could be a mini version of your dad or the complete opposite. You may be thinking about how you might handle your child's first meltdown or their first heartbreak. Embrace these feelings. You are going to be a dad soon. The earlier you start thinking about these things, the better prepared you will be.

Supporting Mom

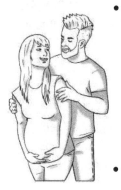

- Mom may not be able to suppress the nesting instincts that kick in, which means she may try to take on too much all at once. Make yourself available for your partner so you are right there if it becomes too overwhelming. For example, she may want to wash all of the baby clothes now, so stay one step ahead of her and relieve her from these tasks so she can rest!
- Double-check that the 39-week prenatal appointment is booked.

Pro Tip: **Practice Those Squats!** – Leading up to delivery day, it's a good idea for mom to regularly start practicing her squats! This pregnancy technique not only helps mom deal with contractions, but also encourages baby deeper down into her pelvis and when the time comes, increases her pelvic opening which helps with dilation.

Reminder: **Early Labor Signs** – Be on the lookout for the early signs of labor mentioned in week 35.

Fun Fact: **Nesting instinct** is a common behavioral trait found in most mammals including humans, and it can also be observed within many other animal species such as birds, mice and squirrels. It is when the expecting mother prepares their home to ensure it is safe and ready for their newborn's arrival. Although mom is likely feeling quite tired by now, she may experience a burst of energy and urge to clean and wash things around the home and ensure everything is prepared for baby!

Did You Know? **Boy or Girl?** – Mom's that are expecting a boy tend to have a bigger appetite during pregnancy than those expecting girls and consequently boys normally weigh more at birth than girls.

Welcome to Week 39
C-Sections & Inductions:
Preparing for Alternative Options

___**TL, DR**___: *Understanding C-Sections and Inductions and where you come into play…*

Important Note:	Check out Chapter 10 for the '3 Stages of Labor and Delivery' ahead of time, so you know what to expect when mom goes into labor - *as it may be before her due date!*

5 minute read

Fast facts covering:

- C-Section Expectations
  - How you can help!
- Medical and Natural Inductions
- 39 Week Prenatal Appointment

A C-Section is major surgery, there is no light way of putting it.

Typically, mom is given an epidural or similar anesthesia. She normally remains conscious and just like a vaginal delivery, can still watch the baby come out. Once mom is numbed and medicated, a horizontal incision is made on the abdomen and another is done into the uterus. The baby is then removed from the uterus and cared for. After the baby is done being checked, the incision is closed up with stitches. Generally, the entire process takes between thirty to forty-five minutes and in contrast to a medication-free vaginal birth, it is usually quick and painless!

C-Sections can occur for a variety of reasons:

- Baby is not facing head down (or in breech position)
- Baby is too big to fit out of the birth canal
- Labor does not progress and the baby's heart rate is in distress
- Vaginal infections such as genital herpes
- There are twins or multiples

You can expect to join mom in the surgery room during the procedure and it is important you stay by her side throughout to provide support and reassurance. Once baby is born, help mom perform skin to skin contact with your baby and even join in yourself by placing baby on your bare chest!

Afterward, however, mom will be in pain from the surgery and probably a bit loopy. This is all totally normal and is experienced by most C-Section patients!

C-Section Recovery

Mom will need a lot of help with everyday tasks if she has a C-Section. She will be unable to lift anything heavier than the baby and the car seat. Even getting in and out of bed will be difficult for her. Make yourself totally available! Instead of her asking if she needs help, just take the initiative and do it.

Some ideas:

- Bring breakfast to her in bed each day.
- Encourage her to walk around at least once a day.
- If mom is feeding baby, have pillows around her to make it easier to cradle baby.
- Help her treat the scar following the doctor's orders.
- Assist in showering and getting dressed.
- Tell her she is beautiful even if getting dressed means throwing on the same pair of sweatpants that are covered in spit-up and ice cream!

Full recovery and healing from a C-Section is generally anywhere from 4-6 weeks, but can be longer depending on the individual.

Types of Inductions

Generally speaking, if there are no signs of labor by around week 42 or there are other complications, your doctor may advise the need to bring on labor sooner to safeguard both mom and baby's health via a 'labor induction'. This can mean a few things, but they usually fall into two categories - Natural and Medical Inductions.

Natural Induction

There are endless ways that mom can try to induce labor on her own. Most women may want to try these methods once they reach 36 weeks, but it is best to wait until at least 39 weeks when your baby is fully developed.

Disclaimer	Before attempting any of the methods below, be sure to consult your doctor first!

Some methods to consider are:

- Walking, a lot!
- Acupuncture or Acupressure
- Sex and nipple stimulation - time to tag you in, Dad!
- Eating spicy food
- Gently bouncing on a yoga ball
- Drinking castor oil (though this one may just lead to a ton of cramping)

Medical Induction

Unless there is a genuine health concern, babies are not usually medically induced any earlier than 39-40 weeks. Some doctors won't even induce until 42 weeks. It really depends on mom and baby's conditions and also your provider. Medical induction may sound scary and if you were to look it up, you may find more negative stories than positive. But it is important to remember, induction occurs for the safety and well-being of mom and baby, so put trust in the process and that your medical team has your best interests at heart.

Some methods of induction:

- **Applying a topical gel of the hormone 'prostaglandin'** inside the vagina in order to bring on contractions and ripen and open the cervix.
- **'Sweeping membranes'** which involves the doctor inserting their finger into the vagina to "sweep" around the cervix promoting hormone release, cervix softening and contractions.
- **Breaking mom's waters** (amniotic sac) using a long tool with a sharp tip or hook, once again inserted into the vagina (sounds painful but usually not). This helps your baby completely drop into the birth canal and promotes dilation.
- **Using a drug called 'Pitocin'** (oxytocin) to encourage contractions. Usually administered via an IV drip.
- **Using a Foley Bulb** which is a long instrument with a balloon on the end. It is inserted into the vagina and the balloon is inflated in order to encourage dilation.

39 Week Prenatal Appointment

Expect to hear your baby's heartbeat and be checked for dilation and effacement if mom opted for this. Be sure to ask the doctor any questions or concerns you may have.

Week 39 Dad's Guide

Baby's Development

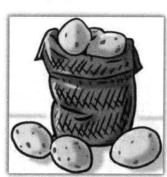

Size Estimate:

- Small Sack of Potatoes (the exact opposite of how you should explain your partners new maternity dress)
- Baby is simply gaining body fat during these last few weeks to keep them warm after birth. Even though they are fully developed, their brain development will still continue for the first few years after birth.

Mom's Changes

Physically:

Recurring Symptoms:

- Backaches, Braxton Hicks (increased intensity and frequency), stretch marks, heartburn, hemorrhoids, swollen hands and feet, trouble sleeping, constipation, dizziness, leaky breasts, itchy belly/skin, and leg cramps.

Emotionally:

- This is a very surreal time for mom. Her due date is approaching, which may feel like more of a 'deadline'. If she does not go into labor by the end of this week, she may be worried and/or feel impatient and just want the baby to come out already!

Dad's Feelings

- All this induction talk might be causing some pressure for you and mom. There is a lingering 'deadline' which you have no control over. The best method is to stay calm during this time and just remember, you waited this long for your baby - you can wait a little bit longer!

Supporting Mom

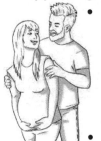

- Mom may want to try out some of those natural induction methods. As long as the doctor approved them, try some with her! Sex and nipple stimulation is when you can make the greatest impact here. Now is your time to shine! Throw on some Barry White or John Legend, toss off those pants and get down to business!
- Double-check that the 40-week prenatal appointment is booked.

Pro Tip:	**Distract Mom** – Mom may be constantly thinking about "when" is it going to happen which can lead to frustration or even anxiety. Help mom relax and keep her mind off things by planning things to do together each day. For example: dinners, movies, relaxing long baths together, gentle scenic park walks, romantic picnics, double dates and sleep ins! Remember, this will be your last week or so as a dynamic duo, make the most of it!

Did You Know?	**C-Sections** – Did you know that around 30-40% of pregnancies require a C-Section? C-Sections are more common than you may think, so don't be too surprised if this discussion point is brought up by your doctor.

Important:

Naturally Induce Labor Safely – It is not considered medically safe for mom to self-induce labor before week 39. Always remember that every pregnancy is different, so you must seek your doctor's advice first on whether it is safe to try yourself and when you can start. If your doctor gives the go ahead, here are a few techniques to elaborate on the points mentioned earlier.

1. Walking – Although not scientifically proven, one of the most popular ways to try and self-induce labor is walking. It can help move baby lower down into mom's cervix and start the dilation process. Some moms swear by this method and it is an easy technique for you and mom to try out.

2. Sexual Intercourse – Many believe that the female orgasm can help bring on labor and start real contractions, sounds like it's worth a shot!

3. Acupuncture – It is thought that this method can enhance blood flow around the body and in turn trigger mom's cervix to start dilating.

Reminder:

Hospital Prep – A reminder to ensure the essentials are ready to go such as – hospital bags are packed and in the car (or next to front door), car has plenty of gas, baby seat is correctly installed, phones are fully charged, pet-care has been arranged etc.

Welcome to Week 40
Past Due Date:
Baby's Cooking A Little Longer

TL, DR: *When you pass your due date, there comes a slew of anxious people asking when your baby will come and mom may have some anxiety about being induced.*

Important Note:	Check out Chapter 10 for the '3 Stages of Labor and Delivery' ahead of time, so you know what to expect when mom goes into labor - *it could be any day now!*

3 minute read

Fast facts covering:

- Fielding Constant Pregnancy Inquires
- Fear of Induction
- 40 Week Prenatal Appointment

If you've hit 40 weeks, then you've hit the point of no return for your family and friends. I like to believe they all do mean well by checking in constantly. They may just be excited about your baby and want to make sure you are both holding up okay.

But, despite their well-meaning reach outs, it may be causing you and your partner some frustration. It's like - if you had the baby, they'd know! The best way to handle these interactions is to give the same canned response to all.

Nope, no baby yet. I will let you know when it happens!

Short and sweet just like your little growing bundle of joy.

> **Pro Tip:** Next time, don't share the due date with anyone. Simply give them a range such as "sometime at the end of August, early September". This will save you a lot of those nagging questions from others.

Fear of Induction

Losing some sleep over the prospect of induction is completely normal. You or mom may have heard stories of induction taking days to kick in and when it does, it comes hard and fast. But there are just as many positive stories as well. A lot of women are induced and their labors are quick as if they went into labor naturally.

Remain positive and lean on your healthcare team. At the end of the day, the most important thing is that your baby arrives safe and healthy.

40 Week Prenatal Appointment

Expect to hear your baby's heartbeat and be checked for dilation and effacement if mom opted for this. Be sure to ask the doctor any questions or concerns you may have.

At this appointment, they may also talk about induction similar to the review from Week 39.

Week 40 Dad's Guide

Baby's Development

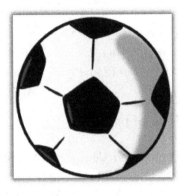

Size Estimate:
- Soccer Ball
- Baby is simply gaining body fat during these last few weeks to keep them warm after birth. Even though they are fully developed, their brain development will still continue for the first few years after birth.

Mom's Changes

Physically:
- Although mom will not be able to feel anything, her cervix is likely thinning out (effacing) and opening (dilating) to prepare for delivery. You will be able to find out by how much during mom's next examination.

Recurring Symptoms:
- Backaches, Braxton Hicks (increased intensity and frequency), stretch marks, heartburn, hemorrhoids, swollen hands and feet, trouble sleeping, constipation, dizziness, leaky breasts, itchy belly/skin, and leg cramps.

Emotionally:
- Mom is probably just done and over being pregnant. The last few weeks are usually just weight gain to help your baby plump up before birth. This can be an uncomfortable time for mom.

it is highly likely that baby will be out by either natural or medical means before this time.

Recurring Symptoms:
- Backaches, Braxton Hicks (increased intensity and frequency), stretch marks, heartburn, hemorrhoids, swollen hands and feet, trouble sleeping, constipation, dizziness, leaky breasts, itchy belly/skin, and leg cramps.

Emotionally:
- Hopefully, by now mom will have gained a whole new appreciation for patience while waiting for your baby to arrive. Some women report feeling much calmer around this time and have settled into the idea of being pregnant without worrying when they will go into labor. Plus, knowing the induction will take place sometime around the 42-week mark gives mom some peace of mind.

Supporting Mom:
- Focus on successful and positive induction stories from others (check Resources section for helpful links). Keeping such a positive mindset on the possible induction will help keep mom (and you) in good spirits.
- Encourage your partner to have open communication lines with you so that you are aware of her needs at all times, leading up to labor and during. Keep her as comfortable and relaxed as possible throughout labor and show her support such as becoming involved in breathing exercise alongside her when it comes time and assisting her to walk around the hospital room, go the bathroom or switching positions in bed.
- Schedule the 42-week appointment.

Did You Know?

Overdue or Not? The majority of babies that make it to weeks 41-42 are not actually late or overdue. This is because in most cases their due dates were not calculated correctly due to various factors such as miscalculations in mom's ovulation cycle, the actual date of baby's conception and dates/lengths of her last period. Only around 3-4% of babies are born on their due dates and some are off by as much as 1-2 weeks! So they really should be called to *'estimated dates'*, instead of due dates! Make sure mom is aware of all this and remind her that it is normal for many women go past their due dates!

97-98% of all babies are born before the end of week 42 – so don't fret, you are still in the normal zone and still have time before baby arrives!

Important:

Strong Contractions – If mom experiences constant contractions lasting from 30-60 seconds and less than 5 minutes apart, call your doctor immediately for further advice.

Pro Tip:

Building Up Mom's Energy - Delivery day is not far away so it is advisable that mom builds up and saves as much of her energy as possible. One of the best ways to do this is a combination of high iron and vitamin C rich foods.

Iron suggestions – red meat, leafy green vegetables, beans and nuts.

Vitamin C suggestions – leafy green vegetables and citrus fruits are your best bets here!

PART 4 - Labor, Delivery and Postpartum Essentials: Let's Get Ready To Rumble!

CHAPTER 10 Learn about:

- **3 Stages of Labor & Delivery:** *navigating through each stage and phase of labor*

- **Skin to Skin**: *take that shirt off, Dad*

- **Baby Care After Delivery:** *everything from circumcision to the APGAR score*

- **Basic Newborn Care:** *get ready for some sleepless nights*

- **Episiotomy Recovery**: *"the husband stitch"...*

- **Postpartum Depression:** *signs to look for*

- **Postpartum Essentials:** *helping mom recover*

- **C-Section Recovery:** *and how it varies from vaginal delivery*

3 STAGES OF LABOR & DELIVERY

Stage 1: Labor Phases

___**TL, DR**___: *Stage 1 of labor happens in 3 phases : Early, Active & Transitional.*

5 minute read

Fast facts covering:

Stage 1 Phases: E-A-T

- **Phase 1:** *Early* Labor
- **Phase 2:** *Active* Labor
- **Phase 3:** *Transitional* Labor

It is usually believed that labor and delivery is simply some painful contractions followed by a lot of pushing. In the grand scheme of things, both are true. But there is a lot that goes on before, in between and after. Becoming familiar with each stage will help prepare you for what to expect, as well as understand why your partner may go from being calm to incredibly tense.

Let's start from the beginning:

Phase 1 - Early Labor

Generally, pain free contractions.

- Normally doctors recommend spending this time at home as it is the most manageable and calming time.
- Now is when you want to start monitoring contractions (see Pro Tip below).

- Encourage mom to eat and rest as she will want to reserve her energy for later stages.
- This is the longest part of labor and its duration can vary greatly. It can last anywhere from a few hours to a few weeks, hence the need to start timing contractions.
- Cervix dilation = up to 3-4cm

Pro Tip:	**Timing Contractions -** You usually want to head to the hospital when mom's contractions follow the 311 rule, meaning they occur every three minutes, last one minute, and continue for one hour long. The best way to monitor contractions is through a 'contraction timer' which you can simply download as a mobile app, allowing you to count from the start of one contraction to the start of the next. Alternatively, you can also jot down the frequency of contractions on paper by referring to a clock or stopwatch.

Phase 2 - Active Labor

Contractions increase in intensity, frequency, and are now painful.

- Consult your doctor for further advice, but generally, when they are 3 minutes apart, you should head to the hospital immediately.
- Mom can cope by using breathing techniques and relaxation methods such as essential oils and music.
- This is usually the best time to ask for an epidural if mom is planning to get one. If so, she is unlikely to experience much pain (if any) for the rest of labor, once it takes effect.
- On average this normally lasts 2-4 hours, but can go longer.
- Cervix dilation = up to 7cm

Phase 3 - Transitional Labor

As mom's cervix prepares for delivery, contractions are more severe, painful and at their peak.

- Mom will most likely not want to talk or sit still.
- Mom can try to cope by moving positions or getting into a warm bath.
- This is the hardest but shortest part of labor and on average takes 10-60 minutes, but can last longer.
- Cervix dilation = 10cm (ready for delivery)

- Offer to hold her hand and breathe through the contractions with her, but follow her lead, as she may not want to be touched at all.

- If she's over heating use a cold damp cloth for her forehead. Or if she feels cold, have a warm compress on standby.

- Have plenty of fluids at hand for hydration such as water or coconut water to replenish those natural electrolytes.

Stage 2: Delivering Baby (Pushing Stage)

_TL, DR_: *Stage two of labor includes your baby moving out of the birth canal and mom may require an episiotomy or may experience vaginal tearing.*

5 minute read

Fast facts covering:

- Pushing your Baby Out
- Possible Episiotomy or Tearing

Delivering Baby

Mom will feel the urge to push and have a lot of pressure in her rectum similar to a bowel movement. Generally, this is less painful than 'phase 3 transitional labor' stage but it can vary.

- If mom received an epidural, she will still feel pressure, but the pain should mostly be gone.
- If an epidural was not used, mom may feel contractions similar to stage one of labor but may also feel an intense burning sensation as your baby's head crowns, commonly referred to as the "Ring of Fire".
- During the pushing process, your baby may be too large to fit out of the vagina. If this is the case, mom's vagina may either tear naturally or, she may need a medical Episiotomy, which is a small cut at the bottom of the vagina in order to enlarge the opening.
- On average the pushing stage lasts from 20-60 minutes. However, for first-time moms, it may take as long as three hours.
- Cervix dilation = 10cm fully dilated

Stage 3: Delivering Placenta (aka Afterbirth)

TL, DR: *Stage three of labor includes the delivery of the placenta. Skin to skin is very important after delivery which is followed by your baby's first health screening and some decisions mom and dad will need to make.*

5 minute read

Fast facts covering:

- Delivering the Placenta

- Skin to Skin
- Baby Health Screening/APGAR Score
- Additional Health Support for Baby

Delivering Placenta

Once your baby is delivered, mom will still need to deliver the placenta, which is a generally painless process

- Normal uterine contractions will continue in order to help push the placenta out after baby is delivered.
- While the placenta is being delivered, encourage mom to perform *skin to skin* with your baby. Doing so provides great comfort, warmth and has a calming effect for both mom and baby. Studies have also shown that it helps to regulate the baby's heartbeat, blood pressure and helps them adapt to life on the outside.
- The placenta is then spread out on a table to ensure the entire organ has been extracted.
- The placenta is generally delivered quite quickly, normally less than 15-20 minutes.

Pro Tip:	**Rip That Shirt Off Dad!** Keep in mind, skin to skin is not just for mom and baby, but for dad too. After mom has skin to skin time with your baby or if for some reason she is unable to, then you should take over for the same reasons mentioned above. Feel free to rip that shirt off, Dad!

APGAR Score

The next step for most babies will be a quick 5-minute health check to determine their condition and if they require any medical attention. This is assessed through an 'APGAR Score' according to the following 5 measures :

1. **A**ppearance (skin color)
2. **P**ulse (heart rate)
3. **G**rimace (reflexes)
4. **A**ctivity (muscle tone)
5. **R**espiration (breathing rate)

Each measure is scored from 0-2, (2 being the highest) with a total maximum score of 10.

Scores are interpreted as follows:

7-10   - Good health. Generally, no intervention is required

4-6   - Below average and may require medical attention

1-3   - Immediate medical attention required

What's Next?

- Baby will be weighed, measured, have their temperature checked and wrapped to maintain body heat.
- You will also notice that baby will get their first shots, which normally include Vitamin K and Hepatitis B. If you would not like these done, you should discuss this with your healthcare team beforehand.
- If you are having a boy, you will need to let the doctor know if you would like them to be circumcised. Since this may be a big decision, you will want to have this discussion prior.

After Delivery: Postpartum Essentials & Recovery

TL, DR: *Recovering from labor and delivery with postpartum essentials such as witch hazel, pads, and numbing spray.*

5 minute read

Fast facts covering:

- Recovering from an Episiotomy and Labor
- Postpartum Essentials for Mom (Vaginal and C-Section)
- Baby Care after Delivery
- Warning Signs for Postpartum Depression

Whether mom had an episiotomy, tore or had a c-section, she will need time to recover. She can expect a large amount of blood loss with the days and weeks following delivery. The best way to recover is for her to rest a lot and ensure she's not lifting any heavy objects other than your baby for the first few months.

After six weeks, there is normally a "six-week postpartum visit" where the doctor will check how mom is healing and decide if she can return to normal activities.

Popular Postpartum Essentials for Mom's Recovery (Vaginal and C-section)

- **Maxi Pads** - absorbs any postpartum vaginal bleeding (aka "Lochia")
- **Ice Packs** - reduces vaginal swelling
- **Witch Hazel Wipes** - reduces the risk of vaginal bacterial infection and relieves swelling
- **Large Cotton Mesh Underwear** - helps air out the vagina and are large enough to hold the maxi pads, ice packs and witch hazel wipes

- **Numbing Spray -** relieves pain

The majority of these items should be provided by the hospital, but you should also have some at home, too.

Additional C- Section Recovery Essentials:

Even though a C-Section does not involve the baby exiting through the vagina, mom will still need the same items as a vaginal recovery. She will also need to take care of her stitches.

- **Scar Cream** - helps to hide the appearance of the C-Section scar
- **Advil (or other)** - pain relief

Baby Has Arrived! Now What?

Well, first off - get ready for some sleepless nights. You will spend the majority of your day and night changing diapers and feeding your baby. It's quite shocking how such a tiny human can eat and poop so much!

The good thing is if they're upset it is usually due to four reasons:

- **Hunger**
    - Signs : baby pecking or putting their hands in their mouth
    - Solution : providing milk for baby (breast or bottle)
- **Exhaustion**
    - Signs : yawning, irritability, and turning head away
    - Solution : snuggling your baby, keeping them relaxed, giving them milk and even a warm bath can all help soothe baby to sleep
- **Dirty Diaper**
    - Signs : fussy behavior and not being able to get comfortable
    - Solution : rolling up your sleeves and changing them!

- **Gas**
  - o   Signs : arching of the back and hiccups
  - o   Solution : burping baby over your shoulder, placing them belly down on a pillow, or rubbing their back in circular motions

Run through this list each time your baby cries to see if any of these will be the solution to calming them.

If baby is still crying after all of these checks, there is a good chance it is caused by:

- **Over-stimulation**
  - o   Triggers - when a baby is exposed to too much stimulation such as bright lights, noises, loud toys, a lot of people - it can cause them to become over stimulated.
  - o   Solution - keeping the lights off or dimmed and reducing noises to help calm them down
- **Colic** (sudden and excessive crying for no obvious reason)
  - o   Triggers - there is no confirmed cause but is thought to be from overfeeding and built up gas
  - o   Solution - laying baby down in a dark room and comforting them with back rubs and patting

What If You or Your Partner Don't Seem Happy...?

It is a very common preconception (and somewhat of an expectation) that once your baby is born that both you and your partner will be just blissfully happy. However, this is not always the case. Postpartum depression is very real but is also very hidden. A lot of parents do not want to reveal they are anything but overjoyed.

It's important to have honest and open conversations with your partner about how you are both feeling and assure each other that it's okay to not feel like you are expected to. If the feelings continue, it's best to talk to a healthcare professional for medical advice.

Important Note:	Please refer to the Resources section for helpful links on Postpartum (and Prenatal) Depression.

Chapter 10 Dad's Guide

Baby's Development

- Baby may resemble Benjamin Button at this time. No, not a young dashing Brad Pitt. I mean when he is a wrinkly raisin of a baby.
- Baby is probably sleeping a ton and eating even more.

Mom's Changes

Physically:

- Mom is most likely feeling pretty beaten up after labor and delivery. This is a very grueling time for her, so she will need to take some time to feel like herself again.

Emotionally:

- She is feeling elated to finally meet the baby! Along with this comes some energy bursts (right before the crash). Continue helping mom, even if she doesn't ask for it!

Dad's Feelings

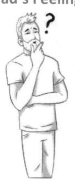

- You are more than likely feeling incredibly overwhelmed. On one hand you have the total joy of seeing your baby for the first time and the complete awe of what your partner just went through. On the other hand, you know this is when the work really starts, and you may have some fear that you can't handle it all. Trust me, you can! I felt the same way after the birth of my first child, but by baby number three I felt like I could raise these kids in my sleep. (haha, sleep…what a distance memory)

Supporting Mom:

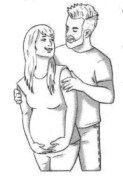

- Make sure mom has all the postpartum essentials for when she is home.
- Practice swaddling to help mom get some sleep at night and keep baby warm.
- If mom (or you) are showing any signs of Postpartum Depression, have open and honest conversations about seeking help and attend appointments together.

Pro Tip:

Colic Rule 3-3-3 – Colic is normally described as extra loud and intense crying (similar to screaming), different to normal crying. If your baby has regular sudden and unexpected outbursts without any obvious reason, then start monitoring this behavior. If your baby cries for a total of more than 3 hours per day, for at least 3 days per week, it continues over 3 consecutive weeks and it is for no obvious identifiable reason, then it is recommended to consult your doctor for further advice.

Reminder:

A reminder that it can take several months for mom's body to fully heal after childbirth before being ready to engage in sexual intercourse again. So keep this in mind, don't be too much of an eager beaver and give her plenty of time to feel up to it again!

Chapter 10 Checklist & Reminders

(Because who has time to make their own list?)

☐   Schedule baby's first pediatrician appointment for the day after you come home from the hospital

☐   Schedule mom's 6-week postpartum checkup

☐   Purchase postpartum essentials

☐   Be a sounding board for mom if she needs someone to confide in with how she is feeling

Now You're Ready To Be A Dad!

Y ou've crushed the last nine months, made it through the forty kingdoms, slayed the dragon, fell more in love with the princess, and are the proud owner of a golden egg.

Prior to reading this book, you may have never heard of an episiotomy, given much thought to glucose tests, or considered interviewing pediatricians.

What felt like an eternity stretched out over nearly a year, may have actually flown by quite quickly. When you look back at the many steps you went through, you could be seeing yourself in a whole new light.

Let's recap:

- One week you morphed into rabbits with an amplified sex drive
- Followed by holding your partner's hand as you wait the agonizing three minutes for the test to reveal those pink lines
- The next, you're holding your partner's hair back as nausea strikes, yet again
- You spent nights awake budgeting for a person who was only the size of a golf ball
- You've sat back to watch your partner pose with a lovable buddha belly
- Put together a crib and installed a car seat that you could have sworn had instructions written in a foreign language
- Sat next to your partner while trying to hold back laughter as you got your first mani-pedi
- Watched your hand cramp as you wrote 62 thank you notes
- Felt your hand cramp a million times worse as it was squeezed to a pulp during labor

- Admired the mother of your child as she labored for hours and still kept pushing
- And finally, you held your baby with a heart so full, it could have filled a stadium

Each week you have been updated on:

- Baby's developments and the best ways to prepare for their arrival, which ranged from detecting your baby's first heartbeat to greeting them for the first time in the delivery room!
- Various ways you can be part of the pregnancy and how you can really make a difference, whether it be helping mom through physical symptoms like nausea and heartburn or timing contractions together.
- The range of emotions you may have experienced throughout the journey that fluctuated from pure and utter joy when you saw the first ultrasound, to downright fear about witnessing your partner in the throes of labor. Not only have you experienced all of these feelings, but I hope to have validated them for you, as they are all totally normal for new Dads.

I hope you were able to close this book, look at your wife, and really understand the world of pregnancy. But above all, I hope you were present in each and every moment and realized that fatherhood starts from the second you discover your partner is pregnant, not once your baby is born.

As you lay awake at night with your newborn baby, ask yourself:

Did you take this wild ride,
from a backseat view,

or, from the passenger side?

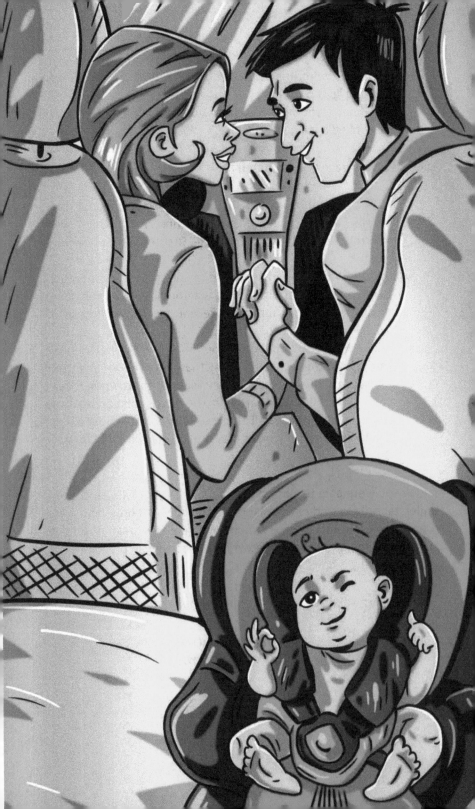

A final message from the Author:

Reviews are not easy to come by.

As independent authors with a tiny marketing budget,

we rely on readers, like you, to leave a short review on Amazon.

Even if it's just a sentence or two!

Simply visit:

A m a z o n . c o m / R Y P

Customer Reviews

⭐⭐⭐⭐⭐ 2
5.0 out of 5 stars ▾

5 star	100%
4 star	0%
3 star	0%
2 star	0%
1 star	0%

Share your thoughts with other customers

Write a customer review ⬅

See all verified purchase reviews ›

We are very appreciative for your review as it truly makes a difference.

Thank you from the bottom of our hearts for purchasing our pregnancy guide and we're hoping you enjoyed it right to the end.

🙏

FEEDBACK

Both Meghan and I would really appreciate your feedback and thoughts on the book. We welcome any positive comments or even any possible suggestions to improve the book for future editions. Please, don't be shy, let us know your thoughts at:

edkinsbooks@gmail.com

OTHER BOOKS IN THE SERIES

In partnership with my co-author Meghan Parkes, keep an eye out for additional books we will be adding to this pregnancy/parenting series over time.

The next instalment of the "Ready, Set ..." series covering your 'Baby's First Year' will be out soon!

If you would like to join our mailing list to be notified of new release books, simply email me at edkinsbooks@gmail.com.

In the meantime, check out Meghan's latest pregnancy book –

'40 Things You Must Do, Before You're Due!' – **It's one helluva read!**

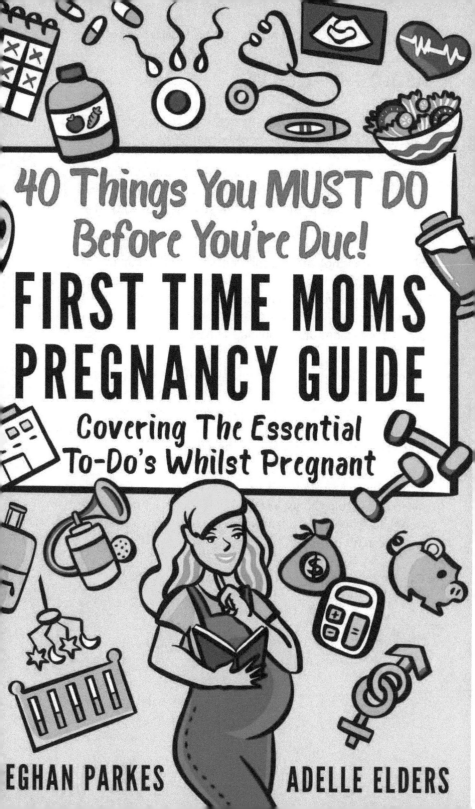

40 Things You MUST DO Before You're Due!

FIRST TIME MOMS PREGNANCY GUIDE

Covering The Essential To-Do's Whilst Pregnant

EGHAN PARKES   ADELLE ELDERS

ABOUT THE AUTHOR

Aaron Edkins is the author of 'Ready, Set ... Pregnant' including the Paperback, eBook and Audiobook versions.

Aaron has received his Masters Degree in Journalism from Columbia University and has also earned the "Father of the Year Award" from his son, which was presented to him on a piece of scrap paper and written with crayon.

When Aaron is not with his children, you can find him partnering with major parenting brands and has written how-to guides for first time dads for several leading publications throughout the US. It is also common to find him answering some of fatherhoods most pressing questions during holiday dinners and group outings.

His humorous writing style coupled with his charming illustrations, uniquely presents fatherhood from a male perspective. If you think to yourself - he won't go there - believe that he will. Aaron completely divulges his own personal stories in a way that helps you feel less alone when preparing to be a dad.

Aaron now lives in San Francisco with his wife and kids. They spend most days arguing about all the family secrets Aaron reveals throughout his books, unknowingly creating more content for Aaron to share in his next book.

Check out his entire parenting book series on Amazon!

ACKNOWLEDGEMENTS

To my loving wife, whose endless support, patience, encouragement and understanding of my personal aspirations as a writer. You made it possible for me to start and finish this book. I am so thankful and grateful for all the extra shifts you have done in order to free up the time I needed to finish this book. A massive thank you and I love you.

To my dearest mother-in-law who also helped support the entire family throughout this long journey, thank you for your continued understanding and for always being there in times of great need.

To my co-author, fellow illustrator and dear friend, Meghan Parkes. Thank you for sharing this amazing journey with me. Your in-depth knowledge and vast experiences have been invaluable and helped create amazing content for this book. I look forward to the release of more upcoming books together and cannot speak highly enough of your current pregnancy guide for first time moms - *'40 Things You Must Do, Before You're Due!' – It's a* must-read!

To our wonderful friend and research assistant Chelsea Doshi. Thank you for the time and effort you have put in this past year to help make this book come to life. You have supported us tirelessly throughout the book's development. Your assistance is always appreciated and everything you do for us is amazing.

Finally, to my ever-growing loyal fan base of readers. Without you, it would not be possible to continue my wonderful writing career and make my dreams into a reality. I feel honored and privileged to have had the opportunity to share my personal experiences and knowledge with you. With this book, I hope to have added some value and entertainment to your own personal journey.

Thank you.

GLOSSARY

- **Afterbirth**: Once your baby is born, the placenta and membranes are then expelled from the uterus.
- **Amniotic Fluid:** Fluid that surrounds your baby while in the womb
- **Amniotic Sac:** Sac of fluid that protects the unborn baby
- **Areola**: the area around the nipple that is slightly discolored
- **Birth**
    - **Medicated Birth:** the use of an epidural during labor and delivery
    - **Natural Birth:** refraining from any medical interventions during labor and delivery
    - **Home Birth:** laboring and delivering your baby in the comfort of your home by either a midwife or doula
    - **Hospital Birth:** labor and delivery while at a hospital under the care of a doctor or midwife
    - **Hypnobirth**: using meditation and relaxation to help a woman through the stages of labor and delivery
- **Birth Canal:** where baby exits the womb during delivery
- **Birth Plan:** a detailed version of events that a mother may put into place to help guide her caregivers on how she would ideally like her labor and delivery to be.
- **Bloodwork**: a series of drawing blood during pregnancy to monitor a woman's levels and wellbeing
- **Bloody Show:** the expelling of vaginal discharge during pregnancy. This can be considered a sign that labor is near
- **Braxton Hicks Contractions:** practice contractions that help prepare a woman for real contractions that occur during labor
- **Breaking of Water:** when the fluid-filled sac around your baby is broken to allow your baby to entirely drop in preparation for birth. This can occur naturally or by a doctor.
- **Breech**: when your baby is positioned feet down in the birth canal. In order for your baby to be born vaginally, it is recommended that your baby be head down instead. This usually occurs on its own as labor progresses, but your baby can

also be flipped this way by mom's movements or doctor's intervention.

- **C-Section (cesarean):** when a doctor removes the baby from the mother's abdomen by means of an incision. This is performed due to: mother's request, doctors' orders, baby being too big, baby's position, or for multiple babies.
- **Cephalic Presentation:** baby is in headfirst position in the birth canal which is ideal for a vaginal birth
- **Cervix:** lower part of the uterus
    - **Cervical Ripeness:** as a woman gets closer to labor, her cervix will begin to thin out and shorten which prepares her for the baby to make their exit
- **Circumcision:** removing the extra skin (foreskin) around a baby's penis after birth by a doctor
- **Colostrum:** the first presence of milk a mother will see when their milk begins to come in. Also known as "liquid gold" as it is the best form of milk for your baby
- **Colic:** persistent crying that a baby experiences which may be due to gas.
- **Conception**: when a woman becomes pregnant
- **Contraction**: the muscles in the uterus tightening then relaxing in preparation for birth
- **Cord Blood Banking:** storing baby's blood from their umbilical cord to be used in the future for certain medical needs such as auto immune disorders
- **Couvade Syndrome (Sympathetic Pregnancy):** when a father begins to exhibit symptoms similar to his pregnant partner
- **Crowning (or Ring of Fire):** the burning sensation felt as baby exits the birth canal and stretches the woman's skin
- **Dilation:** the cervix begins to open and soften during the stages of labor
- **Doppler:** a device used to listen to a baby's heartbeat while in the womb
- **Doula:** an individual (though not a trained OBGYN) used to help guide a woman through pregnancy, labor, delivery, and postpartum

- **External cephalic version (ECV):** when a doctor manually turns a baby into a head-down position
- **Embryo:** unborn baby from week two to week eight after conception
- **Effacement:** thinning of the cervix during pregnancy. The cervix needs to be thinned to 10 cm for your baby to be born
- **Endometriosis:** when tissue grows outside of the uterus as opposed to inside the uterus which is very painful for a woman
- **Epidural:** anesthesia in the form of a shot that numbs a woman during labor and delivery
- **Episiotomy:** a doctor will cut an incision near the opening of the vagina during childbirth
- **Fertilized Egg:** when the sperm fertilizes a woman's egg in order to start conception
- **Fetal viability:** The chances of success for a fetus to live outside of the uterus
- **Fetus:** unborn baby older than eight weeks from conception
- **Foley Bulb (or Balloon):** may be used to dilate a woman's cervix if labor isn't progressing
- **Forceps:** an instrument used to help guide your baby out of the birth canal if it is having a hard time exiting (they look like large tongs)
- **Gestation:** the time between conception and birth
- **Gestational Diabetes:** high blood sugar that is present only during pregnancy
- **Group B Strep Test:** common bacteria in the GI tract that can negatively affect baby
- **Gynecologist (GYN):** a doctor that specializes in pregnant women
- **Gripe Water:** over the counter supplement used to help relieve gas in babies
- **HCG levels** (Human chorionic gonadotropin) – a hormone produced by the placenta
- **Hemorrhoids:** swelling that can occur in the rectum. Generally pain-free, but can sometimes be painful
- **Home Birth** – see 'birth' above

- **Hypnobirthing** – see 'birth' above
- **Implantation**: embryo connects to the wall of the uterus and begins growing
- **In utero:** in the womb
- **In vitro fertilization (IVF):** Combining a woman's eggs and a man's sperm in a petri dish to assist the woman to fall pregnant
- **Induced (or Labor induction):** bringing on labor through natural remedies or through medical intervention
- **Labor:** series of stages that involve contractions phishing baby out of the birth canal
  - **1st Stage:** contractions start and the cervix begins to thin and soften
  - **2nd Stage:** cervix dilates and baby is born
  - **3rd Stage:** once your baby is born and the placenta is delivered
  - **Prodromal Labor (or False Labor):** when a woman experiences contractions and labor pains but labor doesn't actually progress
  - **Active Labor:** six centimeters dilated and contractions begin to get more intense
- **Labor Bar:** a bar attached to a birthing bed that a woman can hold onto during labor to help deliver the baby
- **Lanugo:** light hair covering baby's bodies that protects them whilst in the womb. It may also be present on newborns after birth.
- **Lightening:** when the fetus drops lower into the birth canal in preparation for birth
- **Linea nigra:** a dark line that forms on a woman's belly during pregnancy
- **Lochia**: discharge that comes out of the uterus after baby is born
- **Mastitis:** swelling in a breastfeeding woman's breast tissue that may become infected
- **Medicated Birth** – see 'birth' above
- **Menstrual Cycle:** monthly bleeding

- **Midwife:** trained individual who help women through labor, delivery and postpartum
- **Miscarriage:** when an unborn baby passes away before the 20th week of pregnancy
- **Moro Reflex:** aka "startle reflex". Babies may move their arms and legs in response to being startled
- **Morning Sickness:** the feeling of nausea and act of vomiting during pregnancy that can occur anytime of the day
- **Mucus Plug:** glob of mucus that protects the birth canal during pregnancy that is typically lost as labor approaches
- **Nesting Stage:** during the end of pregnancy, some women have a jolt of energy and an urge to clean in preparation for baby
- **Newborn:** birth to two months old
- **NICU** (Neonatal intensive care unit): a unit in the hospital reserved for newborns with special medical needs such as being born prematurely
- **Nitrous oxide:** 'laughing gas' used to calm mom and relieve pain during labor that is administered through a gas mask
- **NIPT (non-invasive prenatal testing):** bloodwork to test if baby will have genetic disorders (can also reveal baby's gender)
- **NT Scan (Nuchal Translucency):** first trimester test to check for fluid in the back of baby's neck as an indicator for chances of down syndrome
- **Nursery:** room dedicated to baby with a crib and changing table
- **Obstetrician (OB):** doctor specializing in the care of women
- **Ovaries:** a woman's reproductive organ that protects her eggs and releases them for fertilization
- **Ovulation:** when the ovaries release an egg. Occurs once a month.
- **Oxytocin:** used to induce labor and stop bleeding
- **Pediatrician:** doctor specializing in children
- **Pelvic floor exercises:** exercises such as the Kegel that helps strengthen the uterus in preparation for labor.
- **Pethidine:** opioid painkiller
- **Pica:** desire to consume inedible objects
- **Pitocin:** used to induce labor by starting contractions

- **Physician:** a person qualified to practice medicine
- **Placenta:** organ that is made during pregnancy to sustain baby with nutrients
- **PMS (Premenstrual Syndrome):** Common symptoms experienced by women up to 2 weeks before their period which can include cramping, mood swings, headaches and irritability.
- **Postnatal or Postpartum:** the period of time following a baby being born
- **Postnatal or Postpartum Depression:** feelings of sadness (or depression) a mother or father may feel after childbirth
- **Polycystic Ovary Syndrome (PCOS)** – A woman's ovaries may fail to release eggs on a regular basis for fertilization and hence can cause problems when trying to fall pregnant. Cysts can also form around the ovaries which is then referred to as Polycystic Ovary Disease (PCOD)
- **Preeclampsia** – Is a condition that occurs when a pregnant woman's blood pressure increases sometime after 20 weeks. If left untreated, this condition can cause negative side effects such as brain, liver and kidney malfunction.
- **Pregnancy (or Baby) Brain:** a woman's forgetfulness that occurs during pregnancy
- **Premature:** baby born too early before the beginning of week 37
- **Prenatal:** before baby is born
- **Prenatal Testing:** tests done to a woman during pregnancy to monitor baby and moms well being
- **Prodromal labor:** – see 'labor' above
- **Quickening:** when a mother begins to feel baby's movements inside the womb for the first time
- **"Ring of Fire"** – see 'crowning' above
- **Stretch marks:** lines that form on a woman's body due to stretching skin while pregnant
- **Swaddling:** wrapping a baby in a blanket to mimic life in the womb
- **Terms Stages of Pregnancy** – see week 37
- **TL; DR:** too long, didn't read (aka: 'The Short Version')

- **Ultrasound:** doctors use these to monitor baby's growth during pregnancy. It involves the use of high-frequency sound waves to create images that are visible on a screen
  - **Transvaginal Ultrasound:** when pregnancy is early on or baby is too small to be detected by regular ultrasound, a doctor performs an ultrasound scan from inside the vagina
- **Uterus:** organ in the pelvis of a woman
  - **Uterine Lining:** where the egg implants itself and is fertilized
- **Vaginal Tearing:** if a baby's head is too large when exiting the birth canal, it may rip a woman's vagina
- **Vacuum:** tool used to suction baby out of the birth canal if it is too big or positioned in a less ideal location
- **VBAC (Vaginal Birth After Cesarean):** when a woman has a vaginal birth after a c-section
- **Vernix Caseosa:** waxy substance that covers baby's body after birth to provide them with protection
- **Walking epidural:** epidural that allows you to have some feeling in the lower half of your body including your legs
- **Water Birth:** delivering baby in a body of water
- **Womb:** where baby lives before birth
- **Zygote:** A cell that comprises of the combined egg and sperm after a successful fertilization

REFERENCES

Murkoff, Heidi & Mazel, Sharon. (2016). What to Expect When You're Expecting (Fifth Edition). Workman Publishing Company.

Mayo Clinic. (2018). Mayo Clinic Guide to a Healthy Pregnancy. (2nd Edition). Mayo Clinic Press.

Brott, Armin & Ash, Jennifer. (2015). The Expectant Father: The Ultimate Guide for Dads-to-Be (Fourth Edition). Abbeville Press.

Kulp, Adrian. (2018). We're Pregnant! The First Time Dad's Pregnancy Handbook. Rockridge Press.

Oster, Emily. (2014). Expecting Better: Why the Conventional Pregnancy Wisdom Is Wrong and What You Really Need to Know (First Edition). Penguin Books.

Schrock, Leslie. (2019). Bumpin': The Modern Guide to Pregnancy: Navigating the Wild, Weird, and Wonderful Journey From Conception Through Birth and Beyond (First Edition). Tiller Press.

Simkin, Penny. (2018). Pregnancy, Childbirth, and the Newborn: The Complete Guide (Fifth Edition). Da Capo Lifelong Books.

Schrock, Leslie. (2019). Bumpin': The Modern Guide to Pregnancy: Navigating the Wild, Weird, and Wonderful Journey From Conception Through Birth and Beyond (First Edition). Tiller Press.

Borgenicht, Louis & Joe. (2012). The Baby Owner's Manual: Operating Instructions, Trouble-Shooting Tips, and Advice on First-Year Maintenance. Quirk Books.

Greenberg, Gary & Hayden, Jeannie. (2004). Be Prepared. Simon & Schuster.

Dais, Dawn. (2017). The Sh!t No One Tells You About Pregnancy: A Guide to Surviving Pregnancy, Childbirth, and Beyond (First Edition). Seal Press.

RESOURCES

Babycenter.com

Healthline.com

Thebump.com

Womenshealth.gov/pregnancy

Baby.com

AmericanPregnancy.org

Pregnancy.com

Expectingscience.com

Fatherly.com

Pregnancybirthbaby.org.au

Fathers.com

Wikipedia.org/wiki/Pregnancy

Athomedad.org

Kidshealth.org

Fatherhood.org

Mother.ly

Parents.com

Allprodad.com

Miscarriage Support Organizations:

Verywellfamily.com/miscarriage-support-organizations-2371339

Positive Induction Stories:
Kidspot.com.au/birth/labour/types-of-birth/i-had-an-induced-labour-and-i-loved-it

Thepositivebirthcompany.co.uk/blog/category/induction

Birth-ed.co.uk/blog-1/2018/11/1/10-steps-to-a-positive-induction-birth

Prenatal & Postpartum Depression:
Quiz - Babycenter.com/postpartum-depression-quiz

Anxiety & Depression Association of America - Adaa.org

Self-Harm Prevention - Suicidepreventionlifeline.org *(call)*

Self-Harm Prevention - Imalive.org *(online chat)*

Other:
High Risk Pregnancies - Kidshealth.org/en/parents/high-risk.html

Ovulation Cycle - Yourfertility.org.au/everyone/timing

Implantation -
Medicinenet.com/script/main/art.asp?articlekey=19826

Pregnancy Symptoms Relief -
Healthline.com/health/pregnancy/unisom-and-b6

Financial Planning for Baby - Money.howstuffworks.com/personal-finance/family-finance/10-biggest-first-year-baby-expenses.htm

COPYRIGHT

CPSIA information can be obtained
at www.ICGtesting.com
Printed in the USA
LVHW082049220121
676966LV00006BA/305